Multiple Myeloma

It's easy to get lost in the cancer world

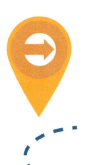

Let NCCN Guidelines for Patients® be your guide

- ✓ Step-by-step guides to the cancer care options likely to have the best results
- ✓ Based on treatment guidelines used by health care providers worldwide
- ✓ Designed to help you discuss cancer treatment with your doctors

About

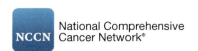

NCCN Guidelines for Patients® are developed by the National Comprehensive Cancer Network® (NCCN®)

NCCN

- ✓ An alliance of leading cancer centers across the United States devoted to patient care, research, and education

Cancer centers that are part of NCCN:
NCCN.org/cancercenters

NCCN Clinical Practice Guidelines in Oncology (NCCN Guidelines®)

- ✓ Developed by doctors from NCCN cancer centers using the latest research and years of experience
- ✓ For providers of cancer care all over the world
- ✓ Expert recommendations for cancer screening, diagnosis, and treatment

Free online at
NCCN.org/guidelines

NCCN Guidelines for Patients

- ✓ Present information from the NCCN Guidelines in an easy-to-learn format
- ✓ For people with cancer and those who support them
- ✓ Explain the cancer care options likely to have the best results

Free online at
NCCN.org/patientguidelines

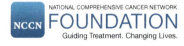

and supported by funding from NCCN Foundation®

These NCCN Guidelines for Patients are based on the NCCN Guidelines® for Multiple Myeloma, Version 3.2022 – October 25, 2021.

© 2021 National Comprehensive Cancer Network, Inc. All rights reserved. NCCN Guidelines for Patients and illustrations herein may not be reproduced in any form for any purpose without the express written permission of NCCN. No one, including doctors or patients, may use the NCCN Guidelines for Patients for any commercial purpose and may not claim, represent, or imply that the NCCN Guidelines for Patients that have been modified in any manner are derived from, based on, related to, or arise out of the NCCN Guidelines for Patients. The NCCN Guidelines are a work in progress that may be redefined as often as new significant data become available. NCCN makes no warranties of any kind whatsoever regarding its content, use, or application and disclaims any responsibility for its application or use in any way.

NCCN Foundation seeks to support the millions of patients and their families affected by a cancer diagnosis by funding and distributing NCCN Guidelines for Patients. NCCN Foundation is also committed to advancing cancer treatment by funding the nation's promising doctors at the center of innovation in cancer research. For more details and the full library of patient and caregiver resources, visit NCCN.org/patients.

National Comprehensive Cancer Network (NCCN) / NCCN Foundation
3025 Chemical Road, Suite 100
Plymouth Meeting, PA 19462
215.690.0300

Supporters

Endorsed by

Blood & Marrow Transplant Information Network (BMT InfoNet)

BMT InfoNet provides information and support services to patients undergoing a bone marrow, stem cell or cord blood transplant service. Our mission is to empower patients and their loved ones with reliable information and support about issues before, during and after transplant so that they may take an active, informed role in managing their healthcare choices. Visit us online at bmtinfo.org, or contact us by email at help@bmtinfornet.org and by phone 847-433-3313.

nbmtLINK

Educating and informing people about their cancer diagnosis as well as the transplant process is an important part of the National Bone Marrow Transplant Link's mission and contributes to the psychosocial support of bone marrow/stem cell transplant and CAR T-cell therapy patients and their caregivers. For information and resources, call toll free at 800-LINK-BMT or email info@nbmtlink.org. The LINK is supportive of resources like NCCN Guidelines for Patients. nbmtLINK.org

Multiple Myeloma Research Foundation

The Multiple Myeloma Research Foundation (MMRF) drives discoveries for new treatments, accelerates groundbreaking clinical trials and fuels the most robust data-driven initiatives in cancer research. Our goal is to find a cure for each and every patient diagnosed with multiple myeloma. themmrf.org

The Leukemia & Lymphoma Society

The Leukemia & Lymphoma Society (LLS) is dedicated to developing better outcomes for blood cancer patients and their families through research, education, support and advocacy and is happy to have this comprehensive resource available to patients. lls.org/patientsupport

To make a gift or learn more, please visit NCCNFoundation.org/donate or e-mail PatientGuidelines@NCCN.org.

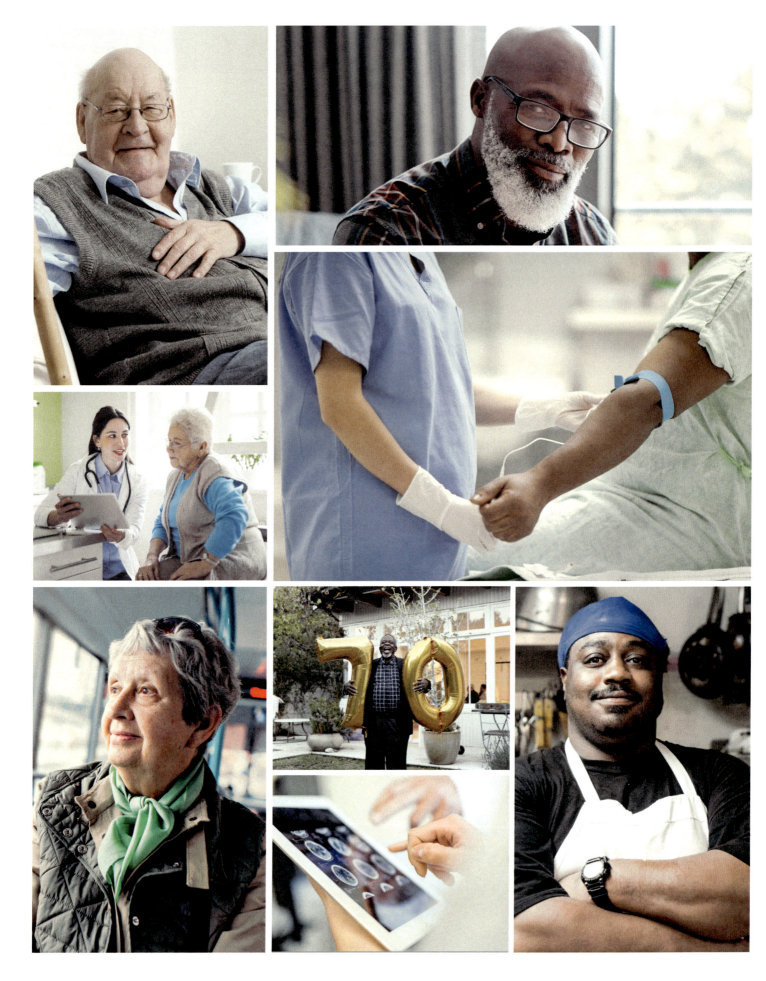

Contents

6   About multiple myeloma

15   Testing for myeloma

28   Overview of myeloma treatments

43   Treatment guide

54   Making treatment decisions

63   Words to know

66   NCCN Contributors

67   NCCN Cancer Centers

68   Index

1 About multiple myeloma

7	What is multiple myeloma?
8	What causes multiple myeloma?
10	Are there different types of myeloma?
10	What are the symptoms of myeloma?
12	Can myeloma be cured?
14	Key points

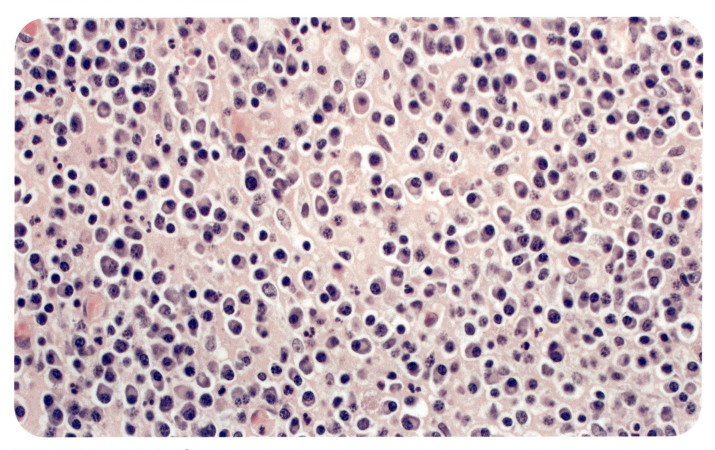

1 About multiple myeloma | What is multiple myeloma?

Multiple myeloma is a rare blood cancer that usually starts inside bones, often causing pain and fractures. While there's no cure yet, new treatments every year are giving people more hope and more years to live.

What is multiple myeloma?

Multiple myeloma (also simply called myeloma) is a rare type of blood cancer that develops in bones and other areas of the body. It results when certain cancerous cells—called myeloma cells—build up in the bone marrow. Bone marrow is the soft, sponge-like center inside most bones. It's where most blood cells are made.

In someone with myeloma, the myeloma cells become so numerous in the bone marrow that they can crowd out healthy blood cells, causing harmful blood problems. This oversupply of myeloma cells also reduces the number of healthy blood cells in the body, which can increase the risk of infections. In addition, myeloma cells release large amounts of myeloma proteins, which can impair bodily functions (like kidney function). Myeloma cells can also destroy bone tissue, causing high calcium levels, bone pain, weakened bones, and bone fractures.

When myeloma cells build up in bone marrow, they can form tumors called plasmacytomas. Rarely, some people develop only one tumor, which is called solitary plasmacytoma. More often, people may have multiple plasmacytomas in different bones or areas of the body, which is why it's called *multiple* myeloma.

What is cancer?

Cancer is a disease where cells—the building blocks of the body—grow out of control. This can end up harming the body. There are many types of cells in the body, so there are many types of cancers.

Cancer cells don't behave like normal cells. Normal cells have certain rules. Cancer cells don't follow the rules. Cancer cells develop genetic errors (mutations) that cause them to make many more cancer cells. The cancer cells crowd out and overpower normal cells.

Cancer cells avoid normal cell death. They can spread to other areas of the body. They can replace many normal cells and cause organs to stop working.

Scientists have learned a great deal about cancer. As a result, today's treatments work better than treatments in the past. Also, many people with cancer have more than one treatment choice.

Older age (age 65 and over) greatly increases the risk of developing multiple myeloma. It's also more common in men than in women, twice as common in Black people than in White people, and two to three times more common in first-degree relatives.

What causes multiple myeloma?

Many people wonder why they got cancer. Doctors don't know exactly what causes cancerous myeloma cells to form. What doctors do know is that myelomas and other cancers often start with abnormalities (mutations) in the cells, which allow the cells to grow unchecked. These types of mutations aren't typically passed down in families (hereditary mutation). They happen on their own and only in tumor cells. Still, you may have a higher risk for myeloma if another family member also had myeloma.

The mutation occurs in the cells' genes. Genes carry the "instructions" in cells for making new cells and for controlling how cells behave. A gene mutation can turn helpful, normal plasma cells into harmful, cancerous myeloma cells.

What are plasma cells? Plasma cells come from white blood cells called B cells, a type of immune cell. Plasma cells fight infection and disease. They do this by making antibodies (also called immunoglobulins [Ig]). Antibodies are proteins released into blood and other body fluids that help your body find and kill germs.

Like other healthy cells, plasma cells grow and then divide to make new cells. New cells are made as the body needs them. When plasma cells grow old or get damaged, they die—a normal and natural process. But somewhere along the line, genetic alterations occur that turn a plasma cell into a myeloma cell.

Myeloma cells, unlike healthy plasma cells, make more and more new myeloma cells that aren't needed and don't die quickly when old or damaged. The myeloma cells continue to make millions of identical copies of themselves. They can spread throughout the bone marrow or grow into a clump (mass) in one or more spots outside of the bone marrow. These masses can destroy the bone around them as they grow.

Myeloma cells, like normal plasma cells, also make antibodies. But the antibodies made by myeloma cells are all copies of a single type of antibody. These are called monoclonal proteins, M-proteins, or M-spike. Myeloma cells make M-proteins without control and not in response to a specific germ in the body. M-proteins don't help to fight infections.

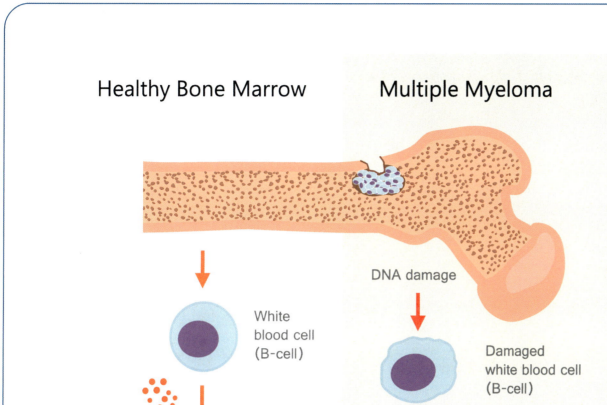

Where do myeloma cells come from?

When antigens (such as germs) invade the body, healthy white blood cells turn into plasma cells, which release germ-fighting antibodies to stop infection and disease (*left*). But in multiple myeloma (*right*), a DNA mutation causes white blood cells to become multiple myeloma cells. Multiple myeloma cells can multiply and spread rapidly. They also produce a lot of antibodies, called M-proteins, which can build up in the bone marrow and cause damage.

Are there different types of myeloma?

There are two basic types of myeloma: active and smoldering.

Active myeloma

Active (or symptomatic) myeloma causes symptoms or affects organs. Common symptoms include bone pain, frequent infections, fatigue, and more. Myeloma that's causing symptoms should be treated.

Symptoms, though, aren't the only signal for treating myeloma. Results from certain lab tests also show when it's time to start treatment. These tests can identify when someone has a high level of M-protein in the bone marrow, as well as kidney problems, bone lesions, too much calcium or too few red blood cells in the bloodstream, and other signs of myeloma.

Smoldering myeloma

When myeloma isn't causing symptoms and doesn't require immediate treatment, it's called smoldering myeloma. People with smoldering myeloma have M-protein in blood and plasma cells in the bone marrow, but usually at lower levels than people with multiple myeloma. People with smoldering myeloma don't need to be treated, but they are tested regularly for signs of multiple myeloma. They can also be considered for clinical trials that explore the benefits of early treatment.

Smoldering myeloma sometimes turns into multiple myeloma. But smoldering myeloma can exist for years before becoming multiple myeloma.

What are the symptoms of myeloma?

The most common symptoms of multiple myeloma are bone pain (often in the back), fatigue, and frequent infections.

Symptoms occur because myeloma cells and M-proteins reduce the number of normal blood cells and normal antibodies. This can disrupt the functions of the blood, organs, and other parts of the body, causing symptoms.

However, some people with multiple myeloma have no symptoms that they're aware of. Their myeloma may be found by a blood or urine test taken during a doctor's visit for something else.

Common symptoms of active myeloma include:

Bone damage and pain

Myeloma cells can cause bone damage when they crowd out normal cells in the bone marrow. Myeloma cells also release chemicals that begin to break down bone. Areas of bone damage are called lytic bone lesions, which can be very painful. Bone lesions also weaken bones, so they may break (fracture) easily.

The most common fracture site is in the bones of the spine (vertebrae). Fractures of the vertebrae can be very painful, although they can sometimes occur without any pain. Other common sites of bone damage from myeloma are the skull, hip bone, ribs, arms, and collarbone.

1 About multiple myeloma | What are the symptoms of myeloma?

Fatigue and feeling weak
Fatigue is severe tiredness despite getting enough sleep and rest. Fatigue, feeling weak, and "brain fog" (having trouble thinking clearly) can be symptoms of anemia. Anemia is a condition in which the number of red blood cells drops below normal, which means there are fewer red blood cells to deliver oxygen throughout the body. Anemia can be caused in part by too many myeloma cells crowding out red blood cells in the bone marrow.

Frequent infections and fevers
Fever is a sign that your body is trying to fight off an infection. Frequent fevers and infections are symptoms of having low levels of normal antibodies and possibly too few white blood cells (infection-fighting cells). A low number of white blood cells can result from too many myeloma cells in the bone marrow.

Bruising or bleeding easily
Platelets are a type of blood cell that help heal wounds and stop bleeding. They do this by forming blood clots. However, too many myeloma cells in the bone marrow can crowd out the cells that make platelets. Symptoms of having a low number of platelets (thrombocytopenia) include bruising or bleeding easily, such as having nosebleeds and bleeding gums.

Thirst and peeing frequently
High levels of M-proteins made by the myeloma cells can cause kidney damage. The kidneys are a pair of organs that filter blood to remove waste. This waste leaves the body when you pee. Increased or decreased urine output is a symptom of kidney damage.

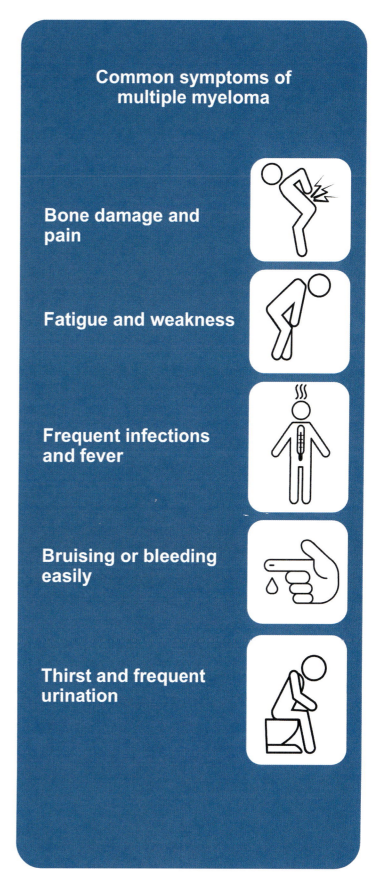

Common symptoms of multiple myeloma

- Bone damage and pain
- Fatigue and weakness
- Frequent infections and fever
- Bruising or bleeding easily
- Thirst and frequent urination

NCCN Guidelines for Patients®
Multiple Myeloma, 2022

Calcium is a mineral needed for healthy bones. But when myeloma damages bones, the bones release their calcium into the bloodstream. High levels of calcium in the bloodstream (hypercalcemia) can also damage the kidneys. Worsening kidney function can further worsen calcium levels, creating a vicious cycle. It can also cause symptoms of extreme thirst, nausea, constipation, muscle twitching, or other related symptoms.

Can myeloma be cured?

Myeloma can't be cured, but it can be treated and controlled for a significant amount of time. New treatments have resulted in more long-term survivors of myeloma now than ever before. For an increasing number of people, myeloma is a chronic medical problem they learn to live with rather than a disease that they die from.

For many people, treatment can keep myeloma under control and reduce or stop symptoms. However, myeloma usually comes back and requires additional treatment.

Standard treatments for multiple myeloma include targeted drugs, immunotherapy drugs, chemotherapy, radiation, and different types of cellular therapy including bone marrow transplantation. Another option is participating in a clinical trial of a potential new treatment.

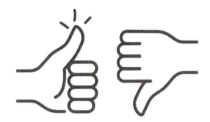

Let us know what you think!

Please take a moment to complete an online survey about the NCCN Guidelines for Patients.

NCCN.org/patients/response

What are antibodies?

Understanding antibodies can help you understand your multiple myeloma diagnosis.

Antibodies (also called immunoglobulins, or Ig) are part of the immune system. They're made by plasma cells to fight infection. Antibodies identify harmful bacteria and viruses, and help the immune system to get rid of them.

Each plasma cell releases only one type of antibody. Each antibody has a different role. The type of antibody made is meant to attack the specific germ causing an infection or illness.

Antibodies are made of two pairs of protein "chains" that are bound together in a Y shape. This includes two identical "heavy" protein chains and two identical "light" protein chains.

- **Heavy chains** – There are five types of heavy chains: IgG, IgA, IgM, IgD, and IgE
- **Light chains** – There are two types of light chains: kappa and lambda

The five different types of heavy chains can bond with either of the two types of light chains. Altogether, there are 10 subtypes of antibodies (immunoglobulins): IgG kappa, IgA kappa, IgM kappa, IgD kappa, IgE kappa, IgG lambda, IgA lambda, IgM lambda, IgD lambda, and IgE lambda.

Myeloma cells also make antibodies, which are called M-proteins. Like normal antibodies, M-proteins are also made of a pair of heavy

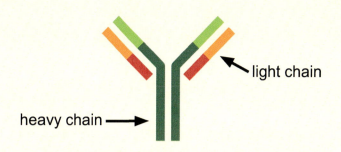

chains and a pair of light chains. Myeloma cells make very large numbers of M-proteins, and most of them are a single subtype. (The most common is IgG kappa.)

Sometimes, the myeloma cells only produce light chains, either kappa or lambda. This results in extra light chains circulating in the blood. These are called free light chains. Some people with myeloma have high levels of free light chains found in their blood or urine.

Knowing your M-protein subtype will help you to better understand your test results. You can follow your M-protein level after treatment to see if it's stable, increasing, or decreasing.

Additional points:

✓ Light chains from M-proteins found in the urine are also called Bence Jones proteins. In about 1 out of 5 people with myeloma, the myeloma cells make only light chains and no complete M-proteins. Doctors call this light chain myeloma.

✓ In rare cases, the myeloma cells make very little or no M-protein. This is called oligosecretory or nonsecretory myeloma.

1 About multiple myeloma | Key points

Key points

- Myeloma is a cancer of plasma cells.

- Plasma cells make antibodies that help to fight infections and play a key role in bone repair.

- Myeloma cells make too many copies of themselves.

- Myeloma cells make abnormal antibodies called M-proteins that don't help to fight germs.

- One mass of myeloma cells is called a solitary plasmacytoma.

- When myeloma cells clump into locations throughout the bone marrow and cause bone or other organ damage, it's called multiple myeloma.

- Smoldering myeloma doesn't cause symptoms or organ damage.

- Active (symptomatic) myeloma causes symptoms by taking over bone marrow. This can result in high blood calcium, kidney damage, anemia, and weakened or destroyed bones.

> New treatments have resulted in more long-term survivors of myeloma now than ever before.

2
Testing for myeloma

16	General health tests
17	Blood tests
20	Urine tests
20	Tissue tests
24	Imaging tests
26	Special tests used in certain cases
27	Key points

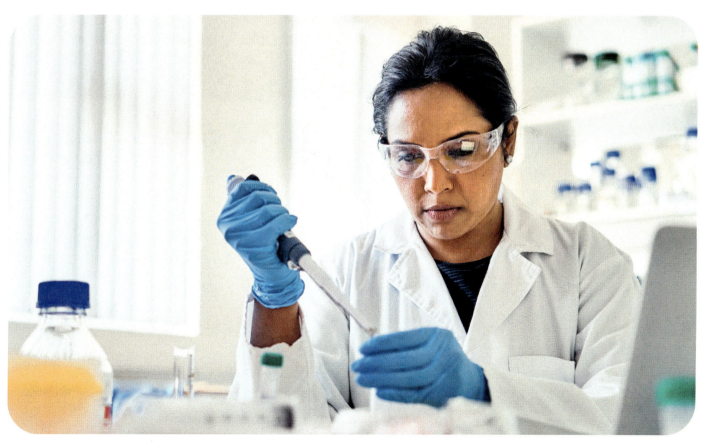

2 Testing for myeloma | General health tests

If your doctor suspects that you have myeloma, you'll need several medical tests before you receive treatment. Some tests check your general health. Other tests are for diagnosing your illness. All of these tests help doctors figure out whether you need treatment and what type of treatment is best for you.

Just the thought of cancer is scary. Having tests for cancer can be scary, too. This chapter will help you know what to expect during testing. Testing will provide a diagnosis, which will help to plan treatment. These steps can help put thoughts into action, which may reduce some of the fear.

Not every person with myeloma will receive every test listed here.

General health tests

Medical history
Your medical history includes all the health events in your life and any medicines you've taken. A medical history is needed for treatment planning. You'll be asked about any illnesses, injuries, and health problems you've had. Some health problems run in families. So, your doctor may also ask about the health of your blood relatives.

Myeloma often causes symptoms, and it's important that your doctor knows if you have them. Symptoms may result from a shortage of healthy blood cells. Or, they may result from damage to the bones or from myeloma cells collecting in certain parts of the body. However, some patients may have few or no symptoms at all.

Physical exam
Doctors typically perform a physical exam along with taking a medical history. A physical exam is a "hands on" review of your body for signs of disease.

During this exam, your doctor will listen to your lungs, heart, and gut. Parts of your body will likely be felt to see if organs are of normal size, are soft or hard, or cause pain when touched. Your doctor will also look for signs of other problems such as bruising, muscle weakness, or numbness/tingling/pain in your hands or feet (neuropathy).

Blood tests

Your blood can tell doctors a lot about your health. Blood tests can reveal signs of myeloma in your bloodstream. Blood tests and other initial tests help confirm (diagnose) myeloma.

Blood is made of red blood cells, white blood cells, and platelets. It also has many proteins and other chemicals. Different types of blood tests are used to measure these different substances in the blood.

Some blood tests are used to assess the extent or amount of myeloma in your body. This is referred to as the tumor burden. Other tests are used to check the health of your bones, kidneys, and other organs. Blood tests may be repeated sometimes to check how well cancer treatment is working and to check for side effects.

For a blood test, a needle is inserted into your vein to remove a sample of blood. The blood sample is then sent to a lab for testing. At the lab, a pathologist may also look at the blood sample on a glass slide under a microscope (peripheral blood smear). Pathologists are experts in examining cells for disease. They can see the blood cells in more detail for a diagnosis of multiple myeloma. They may be able to observe myeloma cells in the blood.

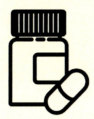

Did you tell your doctor…?

It's important to bring a list of old and new medicines to your doctor's office when you begin testing. It's also important to tell your treatment team if you're using any complementary medicines, especially supplements, vitamins, or herbs. Some of these can interfere with your cancer treatment. Some supplements or herbs can increase or decrease levels of chemotherapy or targeted therapy drugs in your body. This may reduce the effectiveness of treatment or cause more side effects.

2 Testing for myeloma | Blood tests

Blood tests used for myeloma include:

CBC with differential
A complete blood count (CBC) is a test that measures the number of blood cells in a blood sample. It includes the number of white blood cells, red blood cells, and platelets. The CBC should include a differential. The differential measures the different types of white blood cells in the sample. As myeloma cells take over the bone marrow, too few normal blood cells are made.

Serum quantitative immunoglobulins
This test measures the amount of each type of antibody (IgA, IgD, IgE, IgG, and IgM) in the blood. It shows if the level of any type of antibody is too high or too low. An abnormal level of a single antibody could indicate it's growing out of control.

SPEP
Serum protein electrophoresis (SPEP) is a test that measures the amount of M-proteins in the blood. This test is used for both diagnosis and monitoring.

SIFE
Serum immunofixation electrophoresis (SIFE) identifies which type of M-proteins are in the blood. It finds the type of M-proteins by showing which forms of heavy chains (IgG, IgA, etc.) and light chains (kappa or alpha) are present.

Serum free light chain assay
This test measures the amount of free light chains in the blood. In general, the more free light chains there are, the more aggressive the disease is. This test is helpful even when it isn't possible to measure the amount of M-proteins in the blood or urine using electrophoresis. Serum free light chain assay is used for both diagnosing and monitoring myelomas.

Blood chemistry tests
Blood chemistry tests measure the levels of different chemicals in your blood. Chemicals in your blood come from your liver, bone, and other organs and tissues. Abnormal levels of certain chemicals in the blood may be a sign that an organ isn't working well. These abnormal levels can be caused by cancer or other health problems.

The main blood chemistry tests used to help detect multiple myeloma are shown in Guide 1.

2 Testing for myeloma | Blood tests

Guide 1
Blood chemistry tests used to detect multiple myeloma

Albumin	Albumin is the main protein in blood plasma. Low levels of this protein may be a sign of advanced myeloma.
Beta-2 microglobulin	Beta-2 microglobulin is a protein made by many types of cells, including myeloma cells. The amount of this protein in your body usually reflects how advanced your myeloma is.
BUN	Blood urea nitrogen (BUN) is a waste product made by the liver and filtered out of blood into urine by the kidneys. BUN is measured with a blood chemistry test. High levels in the blood may be a sign of kidney damage.
Calcium	Calcium is a mineral found in many parts of the body, but especially in bones. High levels of calcium in the blood may be a sign of myeloma destroying bone. Too much calcium in your blood (hypercalcemia) can damage your kidneys and cause symptoms of fatigue, weakness, and confusion.
Creatinine	Creatinine is waste from muscles that's filtered out of blood into urine by the kidneys. High levels of creatinine in the blood may be a sign of kidney damage. Creatinine clearance is a measure of how long it takes your kidneys to rid the waste product from your blood. This test involves taking a 24-hour sample of urine and comparing it to the level of creatinine in your blood. This test shows how well your kidneys are working.
LDH	Lactate dehydrogenase (LDH) is a protein made by many types of cells, including myeloma cells. High levels of LDH may be a sign of advanced myeloma.
Uric acid	Uric acid is one of the chemicals released by dying cancer cells. Very high levels of uric acid and other chemicals in the blood can be very dangerous. It can cause serious damage to organs such as the kidneys.
Electrolytes	Electrolytes are minerals in the blood that are needed for organs to work well. The electrolytes include sodium, calcium, potassium, chloride, and bicarbonate. Abnormal levels of these chemicals may be a sign of kidney damage.
Liver function	Liver function tests measure the levels of certain enzymes and proteins in your blood. Levels that are higher or lower than usual may indicate liver disease or damage.

2 Testing for myeloma | Urine tests | Tissue tests

Urine tests

Besides blood, urine also reveals signs of disease. Urine tests can be used to diagnose myeloma, assess if your kidneys are working well, and check the results of cancer treatments. Urine tests are also used to assess the tumor burden—the extent or amount of myeloma in your body.

Total protein
Total protein is a test that measures the total amount and type of protein in urine. For this test, urine is collected over a 24-hour period. This test can show the amount of light chains, also called Bence Jones proteins, in the urine. Testing 24-hour urine for protein helps to measure the tumor burden in patients with myeloma cells that mainly or only make light chains.

UPEP
Urine protein electrophoresis (UPEP) measures the amount of M-proteins and light chains (Bence Jones proteins) in the urine. High levels of light chains in the urine indicate a greater risk of kidney damage in people with myeloma. This test is used along with other initial tests when myeloma is first found. It may be repeated to check how well treatment is working.

UIFE
Urine immunofixation electrophoresis (UIFE) is a test that identifies the type of M-proteins present in urine. UIFE is given along with other initial tests when myeloma is first found. It may also be repeated after treatment to check how well treatment is working.

Tissue tests

To confirm if you have cancer, a sample of tissue or fluid must be removed from your body for testing. This is called a biopsy. A biopsy is generally a safe test and can often be done in about 30 minutes.

Bone marrow biopsy and aspiration
Myeloma cells are most frequently found in the bone marrow, so that's where people with myeloma are biopsied. The sample is usually taken out of the pelvic bone (near the hip), which contains a large amount of bone marrow.

This is a two-part test that results in two samples. A bone marrow *biopsy* removes a small piece of solid bone along with a small amount of soft bone marrow inside the bone. A bone marrow *aspiration* removes a small amount of liquid bone marrow from inside the bone.

You may be given a light sedative before the test. Your doctor will then clean the area of skin where the biopsy will be done. Next, you'll receive local anesthesia to numb the area of skin and bone beneath.

Once numb, a hollow needle will be inserted into your skin and then pushed into the bone to remove the liquid bone marrow with a syringe. Then, a wider needle will be inserted into the bone and twisted to remove the solid bone and marrow sample. You'll notice a feeling of pressure as this is happening and you might feel some pain while the samples are being removed. Afterward, your skin may be bruised for a few days.

2 Testing for myeloma | Tissue tests

> If you have a biopsy, be sure to ask if your sample can be stored for future testing.

Lab tests

After the tissue samples are collected, they'll be sent to a lab for testing. A pathologist will view the samples under a microscope to look for myeloma cells. The pathologist may also perform other tests on the samples. It often takes several days before the test results are known. The lab tests that may be performed on the tissue samples are:

› **Immunohistochemistry/pathology review** – This test is used to identify the number and the type of myeloma cells in the bone marrow. A diagnosis of myeloma can be made when at least 10% of the plasma cells (1 out of every 10 cells) in the bone marrow sample are myeloma cells.

› **Flow cytometry** – This test can identify abnormal plasma cells in the bone

Bone marrow biopsy

Doctors use a bone marrow biopsy and aspiration to remove samples of solid bone marrow and liquid bone marrow for testing. These tests are often done at the same time on the pelvic bone.

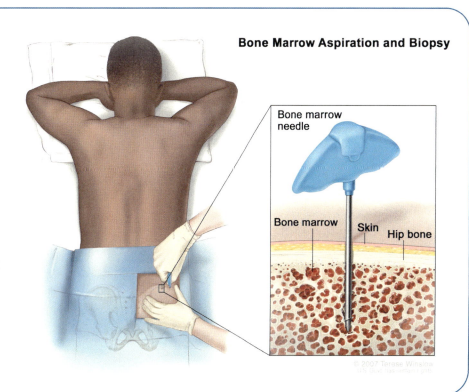

Bone Marrow Aspiration and Biopsy

NCCN Guidelines for Patients®
Multiple Myeloma, 2022

2 Testing for myeloma | Tissue tests

marrow by detecting certain characteristic proteins on the outer surface of the cells. Flow cytometry isn't always done at diagnosis, but might be done after treatment to look for traces of myeloma.

> **FISH –** Fluorescence in situ hybridization (FISH) testing looks for abnormal changes in the chromosomes of myeloma cells. Chromosomes are long strands of genes inside each cell that carry DNA—the body's "instruction manual." Identifying abnormal changes in chromosomes can help your treatment team to better understand your diagnosis and prognosis, and to more precisely plan your treatment. Abnormal changes include deletions and additions to chromosomes, as well as translocations (swapping) of parts between chromosomes. FISH provides one of the important factors to determine whether myeloma can be considered standard risk or high risk. High risk is associated with any of the following:

- Deletion of part or all of chromosome 17
- Deletion of part or all of chromosome 13
- Translocation of part of chromosome 4 with part of chromosome 14
- Translocation between parts of chromosomes 14 and 16
- Translocation between parts of chromosomes 14 and 20
- Copies (duplication/amplification) or deletion of part of chromosome 1

Your pathology report

Lab results used for diagnosis are put into a pathology report. This report will be sent to your doctor. It's used to plan your treatment. A meeting among all your doctors may be helpful for treatment planning once the pathology report is finished.

Ask for a copy of the report. It's your right to have a copy of these results. Ask your doctor to review the results with you. Take notes and ask questions.

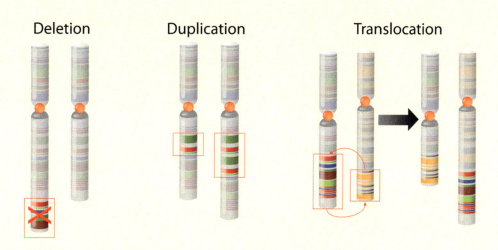

How abnormal changes in chromosomes affect myeloma

Chromosomes are made up of genes that carry DNA, the body's genetic instructions. Abnormal changes in chromosomes can disrupt a gene's function. An abnormality may cause genes to make too many or too few proteins, for example, leading to disease or illness.

Abnormal changes that are important in multiple myeloma include:

Deletion: A loss of a part of a chromosome. For example, a deletion of all or part of chromosome 13 may indicate more aggressive myeloma.

Gain/amplification: A *gain* is when part of a chromosome is duplicated. An *amplification* is when a chromosome is duplicated multiple times. Amplification of a part of chromosome 1 (1q21) is linked with more aggressive myeloma.

Translocation: A translocation is when part of one chromosome breaks off and switches places with part of another chromosome. For example, a translocation between part of chromosome 14 and part of chromosome 20 is associated with high-risk myeloma.

Imaging tests

Imaging tests take pictures (images) of the inside of your body. These tests are often easy to undergo. You'll be asked to stop eating or drinking for several hours before the test. You should also remove any metal objects that are on your body.

Imaging machines are large and may be very noisy. You'll likely be lying down during testing. At least part of your body will be in the machine.

Low-dose CT scan

CT takes many pictures of a body part from different angles using x-rays. A computer combines all the pictures to make one clear picture. The amount of radiation used for this type of scan is much lower than standard doses of a CT scan.

A low-dose CT scan may be used to check the whole body. It can show whether or not lytic bone lesions are present. Lytic bone lesions look as if the bone has been eaten away. These lesions may cause pain and weaken the bones. Since bone lesions are common for people with multiple myeloma, an imaging test such as a whole-body low-dose CT scan is strongly recommended.

PET/CT scan

PET and CT are two types of imaging tests. These tests are often done at the same time. When used together, it's called a PET/CT scan. A PET/CT scan may be done with one or two machines depending on the cancer center.

A PET scan is very good at showing active myeloma and how far it has spread. It can also help show bone damage from myeloma. To create images, a radiotracer first needs

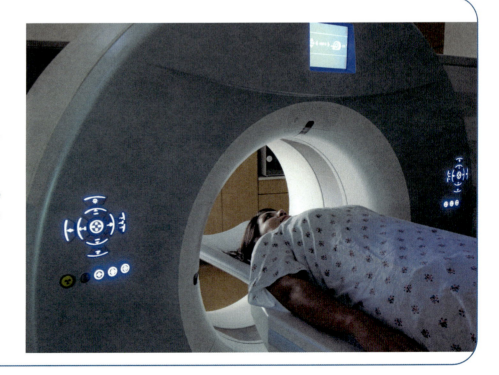

PET/CT scan

Imaging instruments, like this PET/CT scanner, can show what's going on inside your body. During the scan, you lie on a table that moves into the tunnel of the machine. The scan can detect even small amounts of cancer.

to be injected into your body through a vein. The radiotracer emits a small amount of energy that's detected by the PET scanner. The radiotracer makes myeloma cells appear brighter in the images. The most commonly used radiotracer is called FDG. NCCN experts recommend that FDG be used when a PET/CT scan is being done.

Bone survey

A bone survey—also called a skeletal survey—is a test that uses simple x-rays to take pictures of your entire skeleton to look for broken or damaged bones. Bone surveys have mostly been replaced by CT scans, which show bone lesions much better than regular x-rays. However, whole-body x-rays may still be done at some medical centers.

MRI scan

MRI uses radio waves and powerful magnets to take pictures of the inside of the body. It makes images of bone and bone marrow. This type of scan may show abnormal areas where myeloma cells have replaced bone marrow. MRI is particularly useful for telling the difference between smoldering myeloma and multiple myeloma. Unlike CT or PET/CT, MRI doesn't expose the patient to any radiation.

However, these large machines are quite noisy, and you might want to ask for ear protection. The loud, strange sounds in the machine are normal. When you're lying in the machine, it might seem to be very close to your face. It helps to close your eyes and relax while the machine is working. Let your health care provider know if you are claustrophobic or afraid of closed spaces. Your doctor can prescribe a mild sedative to help you relax.

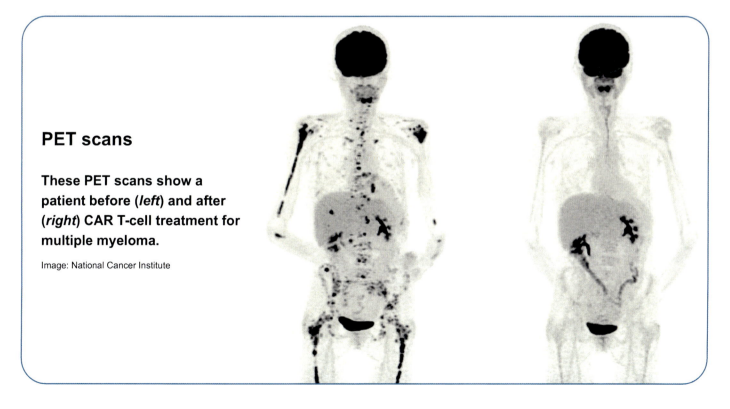

PET scans

These PET scans show a patient before (*left*) and after (*right*) CAR T-cell treatment for multiple myeloma.

Image: National Cancer Institute

2 Testing for myeloma | Special tests used in certain cases

Special tests used in certain cases

Not everyone requires every test. These tests are only used in certain circumstances:

Plasma cell proliferation
This is a blood test that shows what percentage of the myeloma cells are dividing. A large number of dividing cells is a sign that the cancer will grow fast.

Serum viscosity
Serum viscosity is a blood test that measures the thickness of your blood. A large amount of M-proteins in your blood can make your blood very thick—a rare condition called hyperviscosity. Hyperviscosity can lead to neurologic symptoms, headaches, vision problems, bleeding, and damage to your kidneys and other organs.

HLA typing
Human leukocyte antigens (HLAs) are special proteins found on the surface of most cells in the body. The unique set of HLA proteins on a person's cells is called the HLA type or tissue type. All cells in a single person have the same HLA type. This helps the body to tell its own cells apart from foreign cells. It also affects how the body responds to foreign substances.

HLA typing is a blood test that finds a person's HLA type. This test is used to find the right donor for an allogeneic stem cell transplant—a treatment that's rarely used for patients with myeloma.

Echocardiogram
An echocardiogram is an imaging test of your heart. It uses sound waves to make pictures. This test is used to check how well your heart is beating and pumping blood. An echocardiogram is sometimes needed because multiple myeloma symptoms and treatments can affect the heart in some people.

Light chain amyloidosis
Amyloid is a rare protein found in people with abnormal plasma cells that make abnormally folded light chains. Amyloid can collect and build up in tissues and organs throughout the body. The buildup of amyloid, called amyloidosis, can damage organs such as the heart and kidneys. Tests for light chain amyloidosis can be done on a sample of bone marrow, the fat pad (fat from just under the skin of the belly), or an organ that may have amyloid deposits in it.

For many people, treatment can keep myeloma under control and reduce or stop symptoms.

2 Testing for myeloma | Key points

Key points

- Cancer tests are used to make a diagnosis, plan treatment, and check how well treatment is working.
- Your health history and a physical exam inform your doctor about your health.
- Blood and urine tests check for signs of disease.
- Tests of tissue or fluid from the bone marrow are used to confirm myeloma.
- Tests that take pictures of the inside of your body may show bone damage from myeloma. These pictures can also show spots of myeloma cancer growth that are outside of your bones.

Myeloma is a cancer for which we have dozens of available treatment options. If we partner with skilled myeloma specialists to make intelligent treatment decisions, we can expect to live many years of quality life.

– Jim, diagnosed with multiple myeloma in 1997

Hope is a huge part of the cancer process. Because, if you lose that, you don't have the inner strength you need to fight.

– Kris, multiple myeloma survivor

3 Overview of myeloma treatments

- 29 Standard treatment
- 29 Types of different myeloma medicines
- 32 Steroids
- 32 Chemotherapy
- 33 Radiation therapy
- 34 Surgery
- 34 Stem cell transplant
- 36 Clinical trials
- 38 Adjunctive treatment and supportive care
- 42 Key points

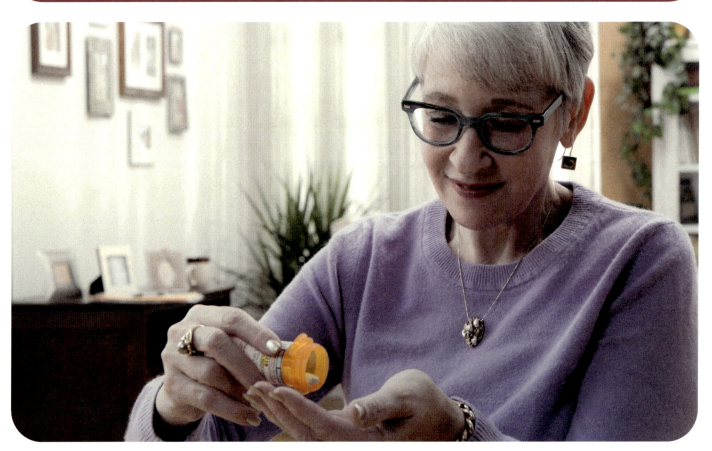

3 Overview of myeloma treatments | Standard treatment

There's no single recommended treatment for multiple myeloma—there are many treatment options. You and your doctors will work together to figure out the best treatment for you.

Standard treatment

Most people with myeloma receive a combination of several treatments. However, no one with myeloma will receive every treatment described in this chapter.

Standard treatment for multiple myeloma often involves a combination of three medicines (sometimes called triplet therapy). For example:

- a proteasome inhibitor
- an immunotherapy drug
- a corticosteroid

These aren't the only treatments for multiple myeloma, though. For example, a chemotherapy drug may be used in place of the immunotherapy drug. Also, the three-drug treatment may be followed by a stem cell transplant or another therapy. Some people even receive a four-drug treatment.

You'll also receive treatment to help relieve the symptoms of myeloma as well as the side effects of myeloma therapy. Participating in a clinical trial of a new drug is another treatment option.

Types of different myeloma medicines

A variety of drugs are available to treat myeloma. Different types of drugs treat myeloma in different ways. See Guide 2.

- **Proteasome inhibitors** block the action of certain proteins (proteasomes) that allow the myeloma cells to survive. Because these drugs specifically target cancer cells, they may be less likely to harm normal cells throughout your body.

- **Immunomodulatory drugs** help to boost specific parts of the immune system against cancer. The immune system is your body's natural defense against infection and disease. Immunomodulatory drugs improve your body's ability to find and attack cancer cells. The immunomodulators used for myeloma also stop tumors from growing new blood vessels.

- **CAR T-cell therapy** is a treatment made from your own T cells. T cells are a type of white blood cell that hunts and destroys cancer cells, infected cells, and other damaged cells. CAR T-cell therapy reprograms your natural T cells to enhance their ability to recognize and target cancer cells.

- **Monoclonal antibodies** are man-made antibodies that attach to proteins on cancer cells.

- **HDAC inhibitors** block the action of histone deacetylase (HDAC) enzymes and may cause cell death.

- **Nuclear export inhibitors** prevent proteins from leaving the nucleus of

3 Overview of myeloma treatments | Types of different myeloma medicines

Guide 2
Drug treatment for multiple myeloma

Generic name	Brand name (sold as)	Type of treatment
bortezomib	Velcade®	proteasome inhibitor
carfilzomib	Kyprolis®	proteasome inhibitor
ixazomib	Ninlaro®	proteasome inhibitor
lenalidomide	Revlimid®	immunomodulator
pomalidomide	Pomalyst®	immunomodulator
thalidomide	Thalomid®	immunomodulator
daratumumab	Darzalex®	monoclonal antibody
daratumumab and hyaluronidase-fihj	Darzalex Faspro®	monoclonal antibody
elotuzumab	Empliciti®	monoclonal antibody
isatuximab-irfc	Sarclisa®	monoclonal antibody
belantamab mafodotin-blmf	Blenrep	antibody-drug conjugate
panobinostat	Farydak®	HDAC inhibitor
selinexor	Xpovio®	small molecule inhibitor
idecabtagene vicleucel	Abecma®	CAR T-cell therapy
dexamethasone	–	steroid
prednisone	–	steroid
bendamustine	Bendeka®, Treanda®	chemotherapy
cisplatin	–	chemotherapy
cyclophosphamide	–	chemotherapy
doxorubicin hydrochloride	–	chemotherapy
doxorubicin hydrochloride liposome	Doxil®	chemotherapy
etoposide	Etopophos®	chemotherapy
melphalan	Alkeran®	chemotherapy

cancer cells, which stops the cancer cells from functioning.

> **Drug conjugates** combine two drugs in one medicine. One drug finds and binds to certain cancer cells and the other drug directly attacks the cancer cells without harming other cells. Belantamab mafodotin-blmf is a drug conjugate that's currently available for multiple myeloma. It's only given to people with relapsed or refractory myeloma after at least four other therapies have been tried.

Side effects of these medicines

A side effect is an unhealthy or unpleasant physical or emotional condition caused by treatment. Each treatment for myeloma can cause side effects. Some common side effects of these drugs used for myeloma include fatigue, drowsiness, weakness, nausea or vomiting, diarrhea, and constipation. These drugs may also cause a low number of red blood cells, white blood cells, or platelets. A low white blood cell count can increase the risk of infection. A low platelet count can increase the risk of bruising and bleeding.

Other common side effects are blood clots, numbness or tingling in the hands or feet, shortness of breath, skin rash, common cold, and muscle aches.

The reactions to treatment differ between people. Some people have many side effects while others have few. Some side effects can be very serious while others can be unpleasant but not serious. Most side effects appear soon after treatment starts and go away after treatment ends. Other side effects are long-term or may appear years later.

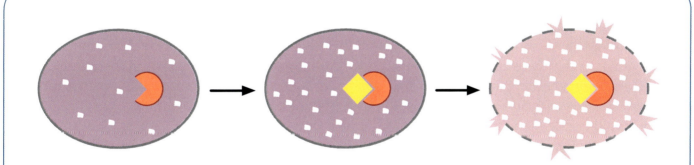

How targeted therapy works: One example

Targeted therapy drugs work in different ways. One way is by blocking a process that keeps the myeloma cell alive. For example, a proteasome chomps up the waste proteins in a myeloma cell. But if a targeted drug blocks the proteasome from doing this, then the waste builds up inside the cell. The myeloma cell becomes overloaded with garbage proteins and is destroyed.

The side effects of myeloma therapy depend on the drug and the dose. Some of the side effects are caused by several drugs but differ in how likely they are to occur. Other side effects are caused by only one type of drug. For example, side effects of CAR T-cell therapy include headaches, confusion, seizures, and a dangerous condition called cytokine release syndrome. This condition's side effects include fever, chills, nausea, headaches, racing heartbeat, low blood pressure, and trouble breathing.

Not all side effects of different myeloma drugs are listed here. Be sure to ask your treatment team for a complete list of common and rare side effects. If a side effect bothers you, tell your treatment team. There may be ways to help you feel better. There are also ways to prevent some side effects.

Steroids

Corticosteroids (often just called "steroids") are used to relieve swelling and inflammation. Some steroids also have anti-cancer effects. Steroids are often used in the treatment of myeloma because of their anti-cancer effects. Steroids can be used alone to treat myeloma or be used with chemotherapy, targeted therapy, or both. Steroids may be given as a pill, a liquid, or an intravenous (IV) injection.

Side effects of steroids
Common side effects of steroids are feeling hungry, trouble sleeping, slow wound healing, upset stomach, and swelling in the ankles, feet, and hands. Steroids also make some people feel irritable and cranky. Changes in mood can happen from day to day. Most side effects of steroids go away after the drugs are stopped. When used for a long time, steroids can lead to weakening of bones, thinning of skin, weight gain, muscle weakness, and increased risk of diabetes, cataracts, ulcers, and infections.

Chemotherapy

Chemotherapy ("chemo") is the use of drugs to kill cancer cells. Chemotherapy drugs kill fast-growing cells throughout the body. Cancer cells are fast-growing cells, but some normal cells are fast-growing, too. Different types of chemotherapy drugs work in different ways to kill cancer cells or stop new ones from being made. Some chemotherapy drugs can also cause damage to your bone marrow.

Chemotherapy is given in cycles of treatment days followed by days of rest. This allows the body to recover before the next treatment cycle. Cycles vary in length depending on which drugs are used. Often, the cycles are 14, 21, or 28 days long. The number of treatment days per cycle and the total number of cycles given also vary based on the regimen used.

Many chemotherapy drugs are liquids that are slowly injected into a vein (IV infusion). Some are pills that are swallowed. The drugs travel in the bloodstream to treat cancer throughout the body. This is called systemic therapy.

Side effects of chemotherapy
Like other therapies, the side effects of chemotherapy depend on many factors. These include the drug, the dose, and the person. In general, side effects are caused by the death

of fast-growing cells, which are found in the intestines, mouth, and blood. Common side effects of chemotherapy are nausea, vomiting, diarrhea, mouth sores, not feeling hungry, hair loss, and low blood cell counts. Feeling very tired (fatigue) or weak is also common.

Not all side effects of chemotherapy are listed here. Be sure to ask your treatment team for a complete list of common and rare side effects. If a side effect bothers you, tell your treatment team. There may be ways to help you feel better. There are also ways to prevent some side effects.

Radiation therapy

Radiation therapy is a type of local therapy. Local therapy treats cancer cells only in a specific area of the body. In myeloma, radiation therapy is most commonly used to treat an area of bone damage that's painful or a plasmacytoma that's causing pain. Radiation therapy is sometimes used as the only treatment for a solitary plasmacytoma (a single mass of myeloma cells).

Radiation therapy involves a large machine that sends out high-energy rays to a specific area. The rays damage the genes in cancer cells. This either kills the cancer cells or stops new cancer cells from being made. Radiation therapy usually requires a series of treatments over several days or weeks.

Side effects of radiation therapy

Side effects of radiation therapy differ among people. Side effects may not occur in the first few visits. Over time, you may have nausea, diarrhea, or fatigue. You may lose your appetite and may even lose weight during treatment. Other side effects occur in treated areas, such as redness of the skin or hair loss.

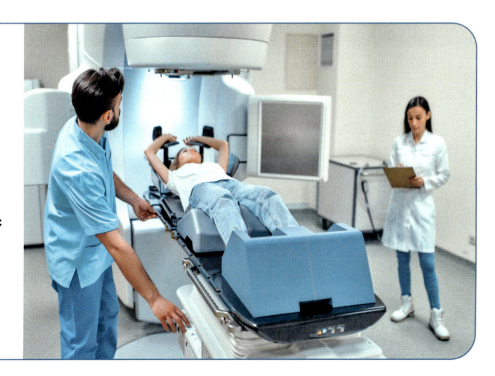

Radiation therapy

Radiation therapy involves a large machine that sends out high-energy rays to a specific area of the body.

3 Overview of myeloma treatments | Surgery | Stem cell transplant

Surgery

Surgery is an operation to remove or repair a body part. Surgery can be used to remove a solitary plasmacytoma located outside of the bone if it's causing symptoms and can't be treated with radiation alone. Surgery is rarely used to treat multiple myeloma, but it may be used to fix fractures in bones or stabilize the spinal cord due to myeloma.

Side effects of surgery

You may experience weakness, tiredness, or pain after the surgery. Other common side effects are swelling and surgical scars. Infections may occur occasionally.

Local vs. systemic therapy

Some of the treatments you receive may be local. Other treatments may be systemic. Here's the difference:

- ✓ **Local therapy** treats only one area or part of your body without affecting the rest of your body. Surgery and radiation are local therapies.

- ✓ **Systemic therapy** involves treatment throughout your body. Chemotherapy and immunotherapy are systemic therapies.

Stem cell transplant

Cancer and its treatment—especially when used in high doses—can damage and destroy cells in the bone marrow. A stem cell transplant replaces the damaged or destroyed cells with healthy stem cells. This is also called a stem cell rescue or a bone marrow transplant. (It's not a transplant surgery like a heart or lung transplant because the rescue cells are given through an IV infusion.)

A stem cell transplant uses powerful chemotherapy to destroy the cancerous cells in your bone marrow. These are restored with healthy blood stem cells, which grow new blood cells and bone marrow over time. Blood stem cells can develop into all types of mature blood cells.

There are two main types of stem cell transplants. An *autologous* stem cell transplant uses your own blood stem cells to regrow bone marrow. An *allogeneic* stem cell transplant uses blood stem cells that come from another person (donor). Allogenic stem cell transplants are much riskier and are now only given to people with multiple myeloma during clinical trials.

Autologous stem cell transplants are a common treatment for multiple myeloma, but they're not for everyone. A stem cell transplant is an intense treatment. Doctors consider many factors when deciding who will benefit from this procedure. Some of these factors include your fitness level, health status, vital organ function, cancer stage, previous treatments, other medical conditions, available supportive care, and additional factors—including your wishes.

3 Overview of myeloma treatments | Stem cell transplant

An autologous stem cell transplant is often performed after other treatments (primary therapy) have already been given.

Collecting the stem cells

The first step of an autologous stem cell transplant is to collect, or harvest, the blood stem cells. Blood stem cells are found in the bone marrow and in the bloodstream. For myeloma treatment, blood stem cells are usually taken from the bloodstream. A few sessions may be needed to obtain enough blood stem cells. You may be given injections (shots) of growth factors beforehand to boost the amount of stem cells in your bone marrow and blood.

High-dose chemotherapy

The next step is high-dose chemotherapy. This chemotherapy is given to destroy any myeloma cells in your bone marrow. But it also destroys normal cells in your bone marrow. This greatly weakens your immune system, leaving you very vulnerable to infections. You may have to stay in a special "clean room" in the hospital, receive antibiotics, or take other precautions to avoid infection for the next few weeks.

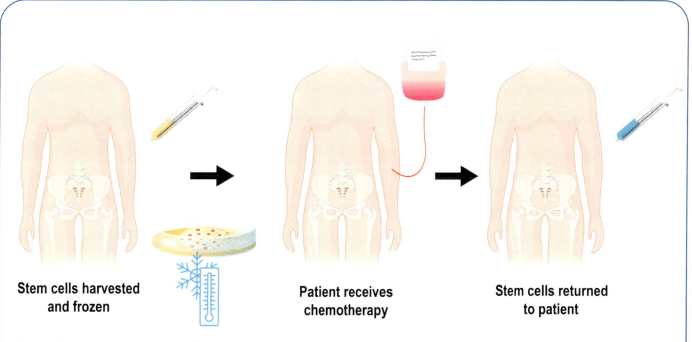

Autologous stem cell transplant

First, stem cells are removed ("harvested") from the patient's blood or bone marrow. Second, the harvested stem cells are concentrated and frozen for preservation. Meanwhile, the patient receives high-dose chemotherapy to destroy any myeloma cells in the bone marrow. Lastly, the stem cells are returned ("transfused") to the patient, where they'll grow healthy new cells in the bone marrow.

Replacing the stem cells

A day or two after chemotherapy, your blood stem cells will be put back into your body with a transfusion. A transfusion is a slow injection of blood products into a large vein. This process can take several hours to complete.

The transplanted stem cells will eventually travel to your bone marrow and begin to grow. This is called engraftment. It usually takes about 2 to 4 weeks for your bone marrow and blood cells to return to minimum safe levels. Until then, you will have little or no immune defense. It may take a few weeks or months for blood cells to fully recover so that your immune system is back to normal.

Side effects of stem cell transplant

High-dose chemotherapy can result in nausea, vomiting, diarrhea, hair loss, and mouth sores. You'll likely feel tired and weak after the transplant and while waiting for the new blood stem cells to grow in the bone marrow. This weak and unpleasant feeling might last for several weeks after you go home, too.

Autologous stem cell transplant is the most common type of transplant used for active multiple myeloma. But it's not considered a cure because the myeloma may come back (relapse) even after long periods of disease control (remission). A second stem cell transplant may be possible for some people who've been in remission for 18 months or more.

Clinical trials

A clinical trial is a type of medical research study. After being developed and tested in a laboratory, potential new ways of fighting cancer need to be studied in people. If found to be safe and effective in a clinical trial, a drug, device, or treatment approach may be approved by the U.S. Food and Drug Administration (FDA).

Everyone with cancer should carefully consider all of the treatment options available for their cancer type, including standard treatments and clinical trials. Talk to your doctor about whether a clinical trial may make sense for you.

Without clinical trials, our treatment wouldn't change. It would always remain the same. Some people refer to clinical trials as receiving tomorrow's best treatment today.

– Jim, diagnosed with multiple myeloma in 1997

Participating in a clinical trial isn't a "last-ditch" effort. A clinical trial is a first-line treatment option for many people with myeloma. Clinical trials give people access to treatment options that they couldn't usually receive otherwise.

Phases

Most cancer clinical trials focus on treatment. Treatment trials are done in phases.

- **Phase I** trials study the dose, safety, and side effects of an investigational drug or treatment approach. They also look for early signs that the drug or approach is helpful.

- **Phase II** trials study how well the drug or approach works against a specific type of cancer.

- **Phase III** trials test the drug or approach against standard treatment. If the results are good, it may be approved by the FDA.

- **Phase IV** trials study the long-term safety and benefit of an FDA-approved treatment.

Who can enroll?

Every clinical trial has rules for joining, called eligibility criteria. The rules may be about age, cancer type and stage, treatment history, or general health. These requirements ensure that participants are alike in specific ways and that the trial is as safe as possible for the participants.

Informed consent

Clinical trials are managed by a group of experts called a research team. The research team will review the study with you in detail, including its purpose and the risks and

Finding a clinical trial

In the United States

NCCN Cancer Centers
NCCN.org/cancercenters

The National Cancer Institute (NCI)
cancer.gov/about-cancer/treatment/clinical-trials/search

Worldwide

The U.S. National Library of Medicine (NLM)
clinicaltrials.gov/

Need help finding a clinical trial?

NCI's Cancer Information Service (CIS)
1.800.4.CANCER (1.800.422.6237)
cancer.gov/contact

3 Overview of myeloma treatments | Adjunctive treatment and supportive care

benefits of joining. All of this information is also provided in an informed consent form. Read the form carefully and ask questions before signing it. Take time to discuss with family, friends, or others you trust. Keep in mind that you can leave and seek treatment outside of the clinical trial at any time.

Start the conversation
Don't wait for your doctor to bring up clinical trials. Start the conversation and learn about all of your treatment options. If you find a study that you may be eligible for, ask your treatment team if you meet the requirements. If you have already started standard treatment, you may not be eligible for certain clinical trials. Try not to be discouraged if you cannot join. New clinical trials are always becoming available.

Frequently asked questions
There are many myths and misconceptions surrounding clinical trials. The possible benefits and risks are not well understood by many with cancer.

Will I get a placebo?
Placebos (inactive versions of real medicines) are almost never used alone in cancer clinical trials. It's likely that you'll receive either a placebo with standard treatment or a new drug with standard treatment. You'll be informed, verbally and in writing, if a placebo is part of a clinical trial before you enroll.

Do I have to pay to be in a clinical trial?
Rarely. It depends on the study, your health insurance, and the state in which you live. Your treatment team and the research team can help determine if you are responsible for any costs.

Adjunctive treatment and supportive care

Adjunctive treatment is another treatment given at the same time as the main (primary) cancer treatment. Adjunctive treatment is given to "assist" the main treatment by improving its safety or how well it works. For myeloma, adjunctive treatment includes supportive care to manage the symptoms of myeloma and side effects of myeloma treatment. It's an important part of overall myeloma treatment.

Here are some ways to treat health problems caused by myeloma and myeloma treatment:

Reducing bone damage
Multiple myeloma often weakens and destroys bones, a condition called osteoporosis. This can lead to problems such as bone pain, bone fractures, and compression of the spine. Medicines are available to help strengthen bones and reduce the risk of bone problems, such as fractures.

Bisphosphonates are one type of medicine that can improve bone health. Bisphosphonates lessen bone pain and help slow down the destruction of bone caused by myeloma cells. They're given as a liquid that's injected into a vein (IV infusion). Bisphosphonates commonly used with multiple myeloma therapy include pamidronate disodium (Aredia®) and zoledronic acid (Zometa®).

A different type of drug called denosumab (Xgeva®) can also help prevent serious bone problems in people with multiple myeloma. Denosumab is given as a shot (injection) under the skin every 4 weeks.

3 Overview of myeloma treatments | Adjunctive treatment and supportive care

NCCN experts recommend that either bisphosphonates or denosumab be given to all patients receiving primary treatment for myeloma. Denosumab is a better choice than bisphosphonates for people whose kidneys don't work very well.

Bisphosphonates and denosumab can cause side effects such as osteonecrosis of the jaw. Osteonecrosis means that the jawbone becomes exposed in the mouth. It's very important to see your dentist before starting this kind of treatment. It's also very important to have good dental care before and during treatment with these medicines.

To help prevent or treat a bone fracture, you may be referred to an orthopedic surgeon. Surgeons can prevent bone fractures by placing a rod to support the bone and hold it in place. Surgery may also be used to treat fractures in the bones of the spine (vertebrae).

Two similar procedures that may be used are vertebroplasty and kyphoplasty.

> **Vertebroplasty** is used to treat compression fractures in the vertebrae. A compression fracture is a break in a vertebra caused by the collapse of bones in the spine. This surgery involves injecting a type of cement into the vertebra. The cement supports and strengthens the bones for pain relief and to hold them in place.

> **Kyphoplasty** is also used to treat compression fractures in the vertebrae. It involves a balloon-like device that's placed in the fractured vertebrae and then inflated. This spreads out the vertebrae to restore the normal shape and height of the spine. Then the balloon is removed

What is supportive care?

Supportive care aims to improve your quality of life. It includes care for health issues caused by cancer and cancer treatment. Supportive care (also called palliative care) is important at any stage of cancer, not just at the end of life.

Supportive care addresses many needs. It can help with making treatment decisions. It can assist with coordinating care between health providers. Notably, supportive care can help prevent or treat physical and emotional symptoms. It can help answer your questions about nutrition and diet. It can put you in touch with institutional or community resources to help you and your family with financial, insurance, and legal issues. Supportive care can also help you find support groups or patient advocacy organizations.

Talk with your treatment team to get the best supportive care for you.

and a type of cement is injected to support the vertebrae and hold them in place.

Bone damage can be painful. Radiation therapy can be used to treat this pain.

Decreasing kidney damage
Myeloma cells cause calcium to be released from the bone into the bloodstream. A high level of calcium in the blood is dangerous for the kidneys. If this happens, you'll be treated with IV fluids and other drugs to help your kidneys flush out the calcium.

Very high levels of M-proteins can cause the blood to become very thick. This is called hyperviscosity. Very thick blood can damage the kidneys and other organs. Hyperviscosity can be treated by a process called plasmapheresis. This treatment filters blood through a machine to remove the M-proteins.

High levels of abnormal M-proteins, including light chains (Bence Jones proteins), can also damage the kidneys. Free light chains combine with another protein in the kidneys. This causes them to be too large to pass through the kidneys. The damage caused by this blockage is called myeloma kidney. Prompt treatment of myeloma is required to prevent permanent kidney damage.

To prevent kidney failure, your doctor may recommend staying hydrated. This means drinking plenty of fluids, especially water. You'll also be told to avoid using certain medications like NSAIDs (such as ibuprofen and naproxen) and IV contrast, which is often given before an imaging test. Your doctor will watch you closely for signs of kidney damage, especially if you're taking bisphosphonates for a long time.

Treating anemia
Myeloma cells may crowd out the normal blood cells in the bone marrow. This can cause anemia—a condition in which the number of red blood cells is too low. With treatment of myeloma, anemia will improve. Sometimes anemia may be treated with a drug called erythropoietin. Erythropoietin helps the bone marrow to make more red blood cells.

Your doctor will measure your blood cell levels at different times during your care. You may also be given a "type and screen" test to make sure your red blood cells won't react to a donor's blood during a transfusion. This test should also be done before receiving treatment with daratumumab.

Read more about anemia in *NCCN Guidelines for Patients: Anemia and Neutropenia – Low Red and White Blood Cell Counts,* available at NCCN.org/patientguidelines.

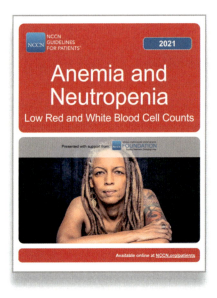

3 Overview of myeloma treatments | Adjunctive treatment and supportive care

Avoiding infections
Myeloma and certain myeloma treatments can increase the risk of infection. The risk of infection can be reduced with vaccines for pneumonia, the flu, and shingles. Shingles is an infection that causes a painful skin rash. Shingles can be a side effect of bortezomib, carfilzomib, ixazomib, and daratumumab. If you're getting these myeloma treatments, you might be given pills or shots to prevent shingles from starting. You may also be given intravenous immunoglobulins to prevent frequent and serious infections.

Preventing blood clots
People with myeloma have a higher risk of forming blood clots in their bodies, particularly in the first 6 months after being newly diagnosed with myeloma. A blood clot that travels to the lungs or the brain can be dangerous, even deadly. Some drugs used for treating myeloma—particularly immunomodulatory drugs like thalidomide, lenalidomide, and pomalidomide—have a greater chance of causing blood clots. If these drugs are used, then you may need treatment with blood thinners or antiplatelet drugs.

Blood thinners are medicines that thin out the blood to lower the risk of blood clots. NCCN experts recommend taking either blood thinners or aspirin (an anti-platelet drug) while being treated with these immunomodulators. This is a complex decision that must compare the risks for clotting against the risks for bleeding, both of which may occur at the same time in people with myeloma. Be sure to talk with your doctor before taking any new medication—even a drug such as aspirin.

Fighting fatigue
Fatigue is a common problem for people with myeloma. Fatigue is tiredness despite getting enough sleep. It may be due to your cancer, your cancer treatment, or another medical problem. Learning how to conserve energy may help. If you're healthy enough, some exercise can also lessen fatigue.

Depression and anxiety
Depression and anxiety are very common in people with cancer. These feelings can be overwhelming. They can leave you feeling helpless and prevent you from taking part in your daily life. Medicine, talk therapy, and exercise are some ways to lessen these symptoms. You shouldn't "tough it out." If you're feeling depressed or anxious, be sure to ask your treatment team for help. Your treatment team may recommend seeing a therapist or mental health professional to help you with these symptoms.

3 Overview of myeloma treatments | Key points

Key points

- Myeloma treatment most often involves a combination of several treatments.

- Targeted therapy drugs are aimed at specific or unique features of cancer cells.

- Immunotherapy uses your body's natural defenses against infection and disease to destroy cancer cells.

- Chemotherapy drugs kill fast-growing cells, including both cancer cells and normal cells.

- A stem cell transplant replaces damaged or diseased cells in the bone marrow with healthy blood stem cells. It also involves high-dose chemotherapy to wipe out any remaining myeloma cells in the body.

- A clinical trial studies a test or treatment to see how safe it is and how well it works.

- Adjunctive treatment for the symptoms of myeloma and side effects of treatment is very important.

Create a medical binder

A medical binder or notebook is a great way to organize all of your records in one place.

- Make copies of blood tests, imaging results, and reports about your specific type of cancer. It will be helpful when getting a second opinion.

- Choose a binder that meets your needs. Consider a zipper pocket to include a pen, small calendar, and insurance cards.

- Create folders for insurance forms, medical records, and tests results. You can do the same on your computer.

- Use online patient portals to view your test results and other records. Download or print the records to add to your binder.

- Organize your binder in a way that works for you. Add a section for questions and to take notes.

- Bring your medical binder to appointments. You never know when you might need it!

4 Treatment guide

- 44 Smoldering myeloma
- 46 Solitary plasmacytoma
- 46 Active multiple myeloma
- 53 Key points

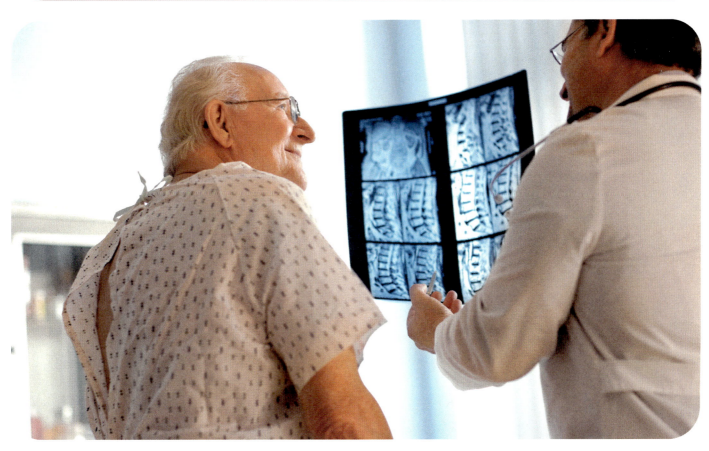

4 Treatment guide | Smoldering myeloma

The previous chapter discussed the many treatment options. This chapter explains how the treatment process will apply to you. Your specific treatment will depend on the extent or aggressiveness of the myeloma, your health, your related symptoms, and other considerations.

There are many treatment options for myeloma. The type of treatment, and when it should start, depends on several factors. Adjunctive treatment and supportive care are also important parts of the overall care for all patients.

Treatment options

The treatment options in this chapter are grouped by the extent of the cancer and the severity of its symptoms. For instance, smoldering myeloma is not considered active and it doesn't cause any symptoms. A solitary plasmacytoma is somewhat more serious; it has one mass of myeloma cells and often causes symptoms of bone pain or fractures. Next, multiple myeloma is when myeloma cells are found in many sites throughout the bone marrow; it can cause a number of symptoms and it requires treatment.

This chapter outlines the treatment process for smoldering myeloma, solitary plasmacytoma, and multiple myeloma.

Smoldering myeloma

Myeloma that isn't causing symptoms is called smoldering myeloma. Smoldering myeloma often takes months or years to turn into active multiple myeloma. For this reason, treatment isn't usually needed right away. In some cases, though, smoldering myeloma is treated anyway if it appears that it will soon turn into active myeloma.

Observation

Observation without treatment is an option for some patients. Observation means that your doctor will watch for cancer growth with regular follow-up tests.

Clinical trial

A clinical trial is a preferred primary treatment option for people with smoldering myeloma. An NCCN panel of myeloma experts strongly encourages people with smoldering myeloma to enroll in a clinical trial if one is open and is the right fit.

Follow-up tests

Many of the tests used for follow-up are the same as those used to confirm active myeloma and assess symptoms. During observation, you should have follow-up tests every 3 to 6 months to check the status of smoldering myeloma to see if treatment is needed.

Progression

If smoldering myeloma grows and starts causing symptoms, that means it has progressed to active (symptomatic) myeloma. From this point, it should be tested and treated as multiple myeloma.

Two main types of myeloma

Active multiple myeloma is defined as having:

At least 10% abnormal plasma cells in the bone marrow or a plasmacytoma confirmed by biopsy

and

One or more of the following myeloma-defining events:

- At least 60% abnormal plasma cells in the bone marrow (that is, 60 or more cells out of every 100 cells in the bone marrow are plasma cells)
- An increased level of calcium in the blood
- Kidney damage
- A low number of red blood cells (anemia)
- Lytic bone lesions or lesions in the bone marrow
- A serum free light chain ratio of 100 or above

Smoldering myeloma is defined as having:

Presence of M-protein in the blood

or

An increased level of light chains (Bence Jones protein) in the urine

and/or

10% to 59% abnormal plasma cells in the bone marrow (that's when 10 to 59 out of every 100 cells in the bone marrow are plasma cells)

and

No other myeloma symptoms or features of active myeloma, such as kidney damage, bone damage, anemia, or increased levels of calcium in the blood

4 Treatment guide — Solitary plasmacytoma

Solitary plasmacytoma

A solitary plasmacytoma is when a person has a single mass of myeloma cells in the body. A solitary plasmacytoma is a type of active myeloma.

A person with a solitary plasmacytoma who has 10% or more abnormal plasma cells in the bone marrow is considered to have multiple myeloma. The following treatment is specifically for people who have solitary plasmacytoma, not multiple myeloma.

Primary treatment

Because there's only one cancer mass, treatment of solitary plasmacytoma requires only local therapy. Local therapy treats a specific area or part of the body, not the whole body. For a solitary plasmacytoma, local therapies include radiation and surgery. Radiation may be given as primary treatment with or without surgery.

Clinical trial

A clinical trial is also a primary treatment option for people with solitary plasmacytoma. An NCCN panel of myeloma experts encourages people with solitary plasmacytoma to consider joining a clinical trial.

Follow-up tests

After primary treatment, people with solitary plasmacytoma should have follow-up tests every 3 to 6 months. Blood tests are necessary at each follow-up visit. Imaging should be done on an annual basis. Other follow-up tests are given as needed. Regular follow-up testing is key to detect signs of progression to multiple myeloma.

Progressive disease

If follow-up tests indicate that the plasmacytoma is progressing even after treatment, then further testing is necessary. This includes all the tests required for diagnosing multiple myeloma.

It's important to know that about half of people with solitary plasmacytoma never progress to multiple myeloma.

Active multiple myeloma

Multiple myeloma that's causing symptoms is called active or symptomatic multiple myeloma. Treatment focuses on both fighting the cancer as well as relieving your symptoms.

There are a number of good treatments for active myeloma—and new ones are being developed all the time. But treatments can't all be given at once just to see which one might work. Instead, your treatment team will first try therapy that has shown the greatest chance of success in people whose myeloma is like yours. This is called primary treatment. If primary treatment doesn't reduce myeloma, then more aggressive treatment will be tried.

Treatments for multiple myeloma

Eligible for stem cell transplant

Primary therapy
- triplet therapy *
- bone-building drug
- supportive care

no chemotherapy

Stem cell transplant

Not eligible for stem cell transplant

Primary therapy/ continuous therapy
- triplet therapy
- bone-building drug
- supportive care

Maintenance therapy

Treatment for relapsed myeloma

4 Treatment guide | Active multiple myeloma

Treatment generally goes along the following lines:

Primary treatment

Primary treatment is the first treatment used to rid the body of cancer. The standard primary treatment for active (symptomatic) myeloma usually includes several treatments given during the same time:

> **Triplet therapy** – a combination of three (or sometimes four) drugs to attack and destroy myeloma cells. A common three-drug combination includes a targeted therapy, an immunotherapy, and a steroid. See Guide 3.

> **Bone-building therapy** – either bisphosphonates or denosumab to strengthen bones and protect them from damage

> **Adjunctive treatment and supportive care** – treatment for the symptoms of myeloma and the side effects of myeloma treatment

The choice of primary treatment medicine depends on whether or not a stem cell transplant might be part of your overall treatment plan. Some drugs, such as certain chemotherapy drugs, can cause severe damage to healthy cells in your bone marrow. This makes it more difficult to harvest stem cells for a transplant. If you're likely to have a stem cell transplant later, then these chemo drugs aren't recommended for primary treatment.

Primary treatment for myeloma also includes adjunctive treatment. Adjunctive treatment is given to "assist" the primary treatment by improving its safety or how well it works.

Guide 3
Primary treatment triplet combinations

There are many triplet therapy combinations. (Sometimes even four drugs are used.) They often—but not always—include a targeted therapy drug, an immunotherapy drug, and a steroid. Your treatment team will consider all your health factors and the status of your myeloma to determine the right choice of treatment for you.

Here are some of the commonly recommended triplet therapy combinations, but others are also available:

bortezomib, lenalidomide, and dexamethasone

carfilzomib, lenalidomide, and dexamethasone

daratumumab, lenalidomide, and dexamethasone

bortezomib, thalidomide, and dexamethasone

bortezomib, cyclophosphamide, and dexamethasone

ixazomib, lenalidomide, and dexamethasone

4 Treatment guide | Active multiple myeloma

For myeloma, adjunctive treatment includes supportive care to manage the symptoms of myeloma and the side effects of myeloma treatment. Adjunctive treatments include:

- Drugs, radiation therapy, or surgery for bone pain
- Drug treatment for high calcium levels
- Plasmapheresis for hyperviscosity
- Erythropoietin for anemia
- Vaccines and treatments for infections
- Blood thinners to prevent blood clots
- Intravenous fluids and possible plasmapheresis to reverse kidney damage

Adjunctive treatments are recommended based on the symptoms and side effects you have. Bone damage from myeloma is very common, so bisphosphonates or denosumab are recommended. Denosumab is a better choice than bisphosphonates for people whose kidneys don't work well.

Drugs such as thalidomide, lenalidomide, and pomalidomide can cause serious blood clots. If these drugs are part of your primary treatment, then blood thinners may also be recommended. Blood thinners are medicines that thin out blood to treat or lower the risk of blood clots.

Other adjunctive treatments may be given as symptoms of myeloma or side effects of treatment appear. You may not need every adjunctive treatment.

Order of treatments

Most people with multiple myeloma receive more than one type of treatment. Treatments are given in the order that is most effective or most needed.

Primary treatment

The first treatment given to try to rid the body of cancer. Also referred to as induction treatment.

Maintenance treatment

Treatment given to keep cancer cells under control after prior treatments worked well.

Additional treatment

Treatment given if prior treatments haven't kept the cancer under control.

Follow-up tests

After treatment has begun, follow-up tests are done to see if the treatment is working or if the disease is getting worse (progressing). Many of the tests used for follow-up are the same ones used to confirm (diagnose) myeloma. For instance, a complete blood count (CBC) will show if the number of any blood cell type is low. Likewise, bone marrow aspiration and biopsy may be done to check if plasma cell levels in the bone marrow have decreased. Other blood tests and urine tests assess if M-protein levels are falling.

Common follow-up tests may include:

- CBC with differential and platelet count
- Serum quantitative immunoglobulins, SPEP, and SIFE, as needed
- 24-hour urine testing for total protein, UPEP, and UIFE, as needed
- Serum FLC assay
- Bone marrow aspirate and biopsy with FISH
- Whole-body MRI, low-dose CT scan, or FDG PET/CT scan
- Assessment for stem cell transplant

Follow-up tests indicate whether the treatment has had an effect. This is called treatment response.

Treatment response

A treatment response is a measurable outcome or improvement caused by treatment. The response is defined by how well treatment is destroying myeloma cells or reducing bone lesions. An improvement in symptoms often goes hand-in-hand with a treatment response.

How well you respond to primary treatment can determine your next step in treatment. A response to treatment may indicate you're ready for a stem cell transplant or maintenance therapy. Multiple myeloma that doesn't respond to treatment is called progressive disease.

Another outcome is when myeloma does respond to therapy (remission) but then comes back months or years later. This is called a recurrence or a relapse. (If a relapse occurs in less than 6 months after primary therapy, the same therapy can be tried again.)

Stem cell transplant

Treatment for active myeloma may or may not include a stem cell transplant. A stem cell transplant isn't a treatment option for everyone. This treatment destroys cells in the bone marrow with chemotherapy and then replaces them with healthy blood stem cells. Your doctor will look at a number of factors to decide if it's the right choice for you.

If your doctor thinks you'll have an autologous stem cell transplant, then your stem cells will be removed (harvested) after four to six cycles of primary treatment, when the number of myeloma cells is low. Enough stem cells should be collected for two transplants. This is done in case you have a second transplant as later treatment.

After the stem cell transplant, the follow-up tests listed above will be repeated to check for a treatment response. Tests to check the level of M-proteins in your blood and urine should be done at least every 3 months.

Maintenance therapy

You'll be offered maintenance therapy after the autologous stem cell transplant. Maintenance therapy is medicine that's given less often or in lower doses to keep (maintain) the good results of prior treatments. The preferred maintenance treatment following autologous stem cell transplant is lenalidomide. Other maintenance options are ixazomib or bortezomib or, in certain high-risk cases, bortezomib plus lenalidomide with or without dexamethasone.

Be sure to discuss with your doctors the benefits and risks of taking maintenance therapy. One risk, for instance, is that maintenance therapy (especially with lenalidomide) slightly increases the risk of developing another cancer.

Continuous myeloma therapy

If you aren't able to have a stem cell transplant, or you don't want a transplant right away, then another option is to continue on primary treatment. With this option, primary treatment is given until no further treatment response is seen on follow-up tests.

More follow-up tests

After stem cell transplant, or during maintenance or continuing therapy, you'll have more follow-up tests to determine whether the myeloma is getting worse or getting better. These tests also check whether your treatments are having any harmful (toxic) effects on your body. Many of these follow-up tests are the same ones as those listed on the previous page.

If tests don't show a treatment response, then you'll receive further treatment specifically for myeloma that has grown (progressed) or has come back (relapsed) after prior treatment.

Relapse

A relapse is when your myeloma improves after treatment, but then your monoclonal protein returns, your symptoms come back, or new symptoms begin. A relapse can happen months or years after your initial treatment. A relapse of myeloma can cause worse symptoms than when the cancer first appeared. Worse symptoms can be a sign of more aggressive cancer. Most people with multiple myeloma can expect to experience relapses.

Talk to your treatment team about which treatment options are available to you. They can explain the combination of drugs and side effects that may occur. Certain drugs are stronger than others and may be harmful to people who are frail or elderly. Some drugs may put you at risk for serious side effects. Some drugs are given only after you've had at least 1 to 3 prior treatments. Your doctors will consider these things, along with the extent of your disease, before deciding on your next treatment. It's important to discuss these factors, and your treatment goals, with your doctors to decide the best option for you.

Progression

Progressive disease means that at least one of the follow-up tests shows that your myeloma is continuing to grow. This growth could be indicated by an increase in M-proteins in your blood or urine, an increase in plasma cells in your bone marrow, or an increase in the number or size of bone lesions.

Having progressive disease doesn't mean you're out of treatment options. Your doctors will suggest trying something new, such as a different triplet therapy or a clinical trial with or without an allogenic stem cell transplant, depending on the timing of a previous stem cell transplant.

Your doctor may also recommend you receive a donor lymphocyte infusion. A donor lymphocyte infusion is when you're given white blood cells (lymphocytes) from the same donor used for the allogeneic stem cell transplant.

If tests show progressive disease during or after additional treatment, then palliative care may also be recommended. Palliative care is given to relieve the symptoms of cancer and the side effects of cancer treatment. It doesn't aim to treat the cancer, but aims to improve your quality of life.

Clinical trial

A clinical trial is a treatment option for many people with multiple myeloma. Clinical trials give people access to treatment options that they couldn't usually receive otherwise. Ask your treatment team how to join a clinical trial. Joining a clinical trial becomes ever more important in a person with relapsed myeloma.

Observation

Medical treatment for multiple myeloma is generally advised. However, observation may be a better or safer option for some people. Observation means your doctors will keep an eye on your condition by giving you regular tests over time. No treatment is given unless symptoms appear or your condition changes.

Survivorship

Survivorship focuses on the health and wellbeing of a person with cancer from diagnosis until the end of life. This includes the physical, mental, emotional, social, and financial effects of cancer that begin at diagnosis, continue through treatment, and arise afterward. Survivorship also includes concerns about follow-up care, late effects of treatment, cancer recurrence, and quality of life. Support from family members, friends, and caregivers is also an important part of survivorship.

Read more about survivorship in *NCCN Guidelines for Patients: Survivorship Care for Healthy Living* and *Survivorship Care for Cancer-Related Late and Long-Term Effects*, available at NCCN.org/patientguidelines.

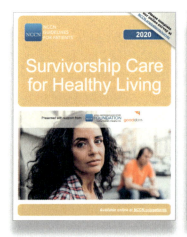
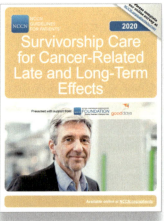

Key points

- Treatment for smoldering myeloma isn't needed right away because it doesn't show symptoms and often takes months or years to turn into active multiple myeloma.

- Treatment of solitary plasmacytoma usually requires only local therapy to treat the single cancer mass.

- Treatment of active multiple myeloma focuses on fighting the cancer as well as relieving symptoms.

- The choice of drugs used for primary treatment of multiple myeloma depends on whether a stem cell transplant might be part of the overall treatment plan.

- Adjunctive treatment of multiple myeloma includes supportive care to manage myeloma symptoms and side effects of treatment.

- Maintenance therapy is given less frequently or in lower doses than primary therapy. Its goal is to keep up the good results of previous treatment.

- A relapse is when symptoms come back or new symptoms begin after a period of improvement.

- Most people with multiple myeloma should expect to have relapses.

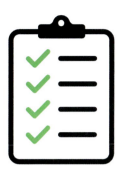

We want your feedback!

Our goal is to provide helpful and easy-to-understand information on cancer.

Take our survey to let us know what we got right and what we could do better:

NCCN.org/patients/feedback

5　Making treatment decisions

55　**It's your choice**
57　**Questions to ask your doctors**
61　**Online resources**

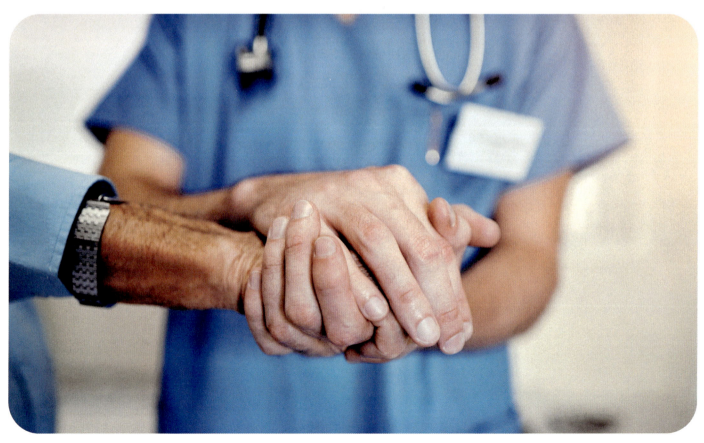

5 Making treatment decisions | It's your choice

It's important to be comfortable with the treatment you choose. This choice starts with having an open and honest conversation with your doctors.

It's your choice

In shared decision-making, you and your doctors share information, discuss the options, and agree on a treatment plan. It starts with an open and honest conversation between you and your doctor.

Treatment decisions are very personal. What's important to you may not be important to someone else.

Some things that may play a role in your decision-making:

- What you want and how that might differ from what others want
- Availability of clinical trials in your area
- Your religious and spiritual beliefs
- Your feelings about certain treatments like surgery or chemotherapy
- Your feelings about pain or side effects such as nausea and vomiting
- Cost of treatment, travel to treatment centers, and time away from work
- Quality of life and length of life
- How active you are and the activities that are important to you

Think about what you want from treatment. Discuss openly the risks and benefits of specific treatments and procedures. Weigh options and share concerns with your doctor. If you make the effort to build a relationship with your doctor, it will help you feel supported when considering options and making treatment decisions. Learning about myeloma will help you make better treatment decisions as you talk with your doctor.

Deciding on your treatment options

Choosing your treatment is a very important decision. It can affect your length and quality of life. But deciding which treatment option is best can be hard. Doctors from different fields of medicine may have different opinions on which option is best for you. This can be very confusing. Also, your spouse, partner, or family members may disagree with which option you want. That can be stressful. In some cases, one option hasn't been shown to work better than another.

Here are some ways to help you decide on treatment.

Second opinion

People with cancer often want to get treated as soon as possible. They want to make their cancer go away before it grows any further. While cancer can't be ignored, there is usually enough time to think about and choose which option is best for you.

You may completely trust your doctor, but a second opinion about which option is best can help. A second opinion is when another doctor reviews your test results and suggests a treatment plan. Copies of the pathology report, imaging, and other test results need to be sent to the doctor giving the second opinion. Some people feel uneasy asking for copies from their doctors. However, a second opinion is a normal part of cancer care and most doctors are very comfortable helping you to get a second opinion. Even doctors get second opinions!

Some health plans require a second opinion. If your health plan doesn't cover the cost of a second opinion, you have the choice of paying for it yourself.

If the two opinions are the same, you may feel more at peace about treatment. If the two opinions differ, think about getting a third opinion. A third opinion may help you decide between your options. It's your cancer, and the decision about which treatment is best is your decision.

Things you can do to prepare for a second opinion:

> Check with your insurance company about its rules on second opinions. There may be out-of-pocket costs to see doctors who aren't part of your insurance plan.

> Make plans to have copies of all your records sent to the doctor you will see for your second opinion.

Compare benefits and downsides
Every option has benefits and downsides. Consider both when deciding which option is best for you. Talking to others can help identify benefits and downsides you haven't thought of. Scoring each factor from 0 to 10 can also help because some factors may be more important to you than others.

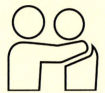

Get group support

Many people with cancer find a lot of value in a support group. In support groups, you can ask questions and hear about the experiences of other people with cancer. Some people may be newly diagnosed, while others may be finished with treatment.

A support group can help with emotional and psychological needs. A support group can also be a good source of practical advice and helpful tips. People with common ground can share information on their experiences, financial and emotional burdens, coping strategies, and knowledge about research and treatments.

Ask your doctors or supportive care team about finding a myeloma or cancer support community. Support groups can be found online and in-person groups are often available in larger communities.

Questions to ask your doctors

Possible questions to ask your doctors are listed on the following pages. Feel free to use these questions or come up with your own. Be clear about your goals for treatment and find out what to expect from treatment.

Questions to ask about testing and staging

1. What type of myeloma do I have?

2. Can it be cured? If not, how well can treatment stop it from growing?

3. What tests will I have?

4. How do I prepare for testing?

5. When will I have a biopsy? Will I have more than one? What are the risks? Is it painful?

6. Where do I go to get tested? How long will the tests take? Will any test hurt?

7. What if I'm pregnant or planning to get pregnant?

8. How often are these tests wrong?

9. Should I bring someone with me?

10. Should I bring a list of my medications?

11. How soon will I know the results and who will explain them to me?

12. Would you give me a copy of the pathology report and other test results?

13. Will my tumor or biopsy tissue be saved for further testing? Can I have it sent to another facility for additional testing?

14. Who will talk with me about the next steps? When?

15. Who can I call if I need help immediately?

5 Making treatment decisions | Questions to ask your doctors

Questions to ask about treatment options

1. What are my treatment options? Are you suggesting options from the NCCN Guidelines, or have you modified the standard approach in my situation?

2. Do your suggested options include clinical trials? Please explain why.

3. How many patients like me have you treated?

4. Will the treatment hurt?

5. What will happen if I do nothing?

6. How do my age, overall health, and other factors affect my options?

7. Does any option offer a cure or long-term cancer control? Are my chances any better for one option than another? Less time-consuming? Less expensive?

8. How do you know if my treatment is working?

9. How will I know if my treatment is working, and how long does it usually take?

10. What are my options if treatment stops working?

11. What are the possible complications? What are the short- and long-term side effects of treatment?

12. How will treatment affect me? Will my sense of smell or taste change? Will my hair fall out?

13. How soon will I need to make my treatment decisions?

14. What can be done to prevent or relieve the side effects of treatment?

15. What supportive care services are available to me during and after treatment?

16. Can I stop treatment at any time? What will happen if I stop treatment?

5 Making treatment decisions | Questions to ask your doctors

Questions to ask about getting treatment

1. Do I have to go to the hospital or elsewhere? How often? How long is each visit?

2. What do I need to think about if I have to travel for treatment?

3. Do I have a choice of when to begin treatment? Can I choose the days and times of treatment?

4. How do I prepare for treatment? Do I have to stop taking any of my medicines? Are there foods I should avoid?

5. Should I bring someone with me when I get treated?

6. How much will the treatment cost me? What does my insurance cover? Are there any grants available to me? Would a clinical trial provide some medications for free?

7. Will I miss work or school? Will I be able to drive?

8. Who do I call when you're off duty? Should I go to the emergency room?

9. Is home care after treatment needed? If yes, what type?

10. Will I be able to manage my own health?

11. Will I be able to return to my normal activities? If so, when?

12. What emotional and psychological help is available for me and for those taking care of me?

5 Making treatment decisions | Questions to ask your doctors

Questions to ask about clinical trials

1. Are there clinical trials for my type of myeloma?

2. What are the treatments used in the clinical trial?

3. What does the treatment do?

4. Has the treatment been used before? Has it been used for other types of cancer?

5. What are the risks and benefits of joining the clinical trial and the treatment being tested?

6. Will the trial need a biopsy sample?

7. What side effects should I expect? How will the side effects be controlled?

8. How long will I be in the clinical trial?

9. Will I be able to get other treatment if this doesn't work?

10. How will you know if the treatment is working?

11. Will the clinical trial cost me anything? If so, how much?

Online resources

American Cancer Society
cancer.org/cancer/multiple-myeloma.html

Blood & Marrow Transplant Information Network (BMT InfoNet)
bmtinfonet.org

International Myeloma Foundation
myeloma.org

Leukemia & Lymphoma Society
lls.org/myeloma/myeloma-overview

Multiple Myeloma Research Foundation
themmrf.org

National Bone Marrow Transplant Link (nbmtLINK)
nbmtlink.org

National Cancer Institute
cancer.gov/types/myeloma

National Coalition for Cancer Survivorship
canceradvocacy.org

NCCN Patient and Caregiver Resources
nccn.org/patientresources/patient-resources/support-for-patients-caregivers

Standing in the Gaap (for African Americans living with multiple myeloma)
myelomacentral.com/multiple-myeloma-african-americans/

The Myeloma Crowd
myelomacrowd.org

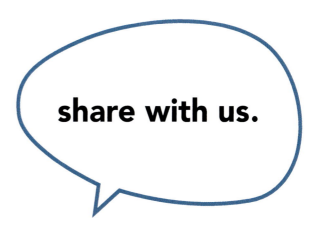

Take our survey
And help make the NCCN Guidelines for Patients better for everyone!

NCCN.org/patients/comments

Words to know

active (symptomatic) myeloma
When abnormal plasma cells (myeloma cells) have increased in the bone marrow and are causing symptoms such as kidney problems and bone damage.

adjunctive treatment
Medicine for symptoms of myeloma and for side effects of treatment that's given at the same time as the main cancer treatment.

allogeneic stem cell transplant
A treatment that destroys cells in the bone marrow with chemotherapy and then replaces them with healthy blood stem cells from another person (donor). Rarely used for multiple myeloma therapy.

amyloidosis
A health condition in which a protein called amyloid builds up in and damages organs.

anemia
A health condition in which the number of red blood cells is low.

antibody
A protein made by plasma cells to help fight off infections. Also called immunoglobulin.

aspiration
A procedure that removes a small amount of liquid bone marrow to be tested for a disease.

asymptomatic
Having no signs or symptoms of disease.

autologous stem cell transplant
A treatment that destroys cells in the bone marrow with chemotherapy and then replaces them with your own healthy blood stem cells.

B cell
A type of white blood cell that turns into a plasma cell in response to germs.

Bence Jones protein
The shorter protein chain (free light chain) that is part of an M-protein and found in the urine.

biopsy
A procedure that removes fluid or tissue samples to be tested for a disease.

bisphosphonates
Drugs that help improve bone strength and prevent loss of bone mass.

blood stem cell
An immature cell from which all other types of blood cells are made.

bone lesion
An area of bone damage or abnormal tissue in the bone.

bone marrow
The soft, sponge-like tissue in the center of most bones where blood cells are made.

chemotherapy
Cancer drugs that stop the cell life cycle so cells don't increase in number.

chromosomes
The structures within cells that contain coded instructions for cell behavior.

clinical trial
A type of research that assesses how well health tests or treatments work in people.

complete blood count (CBC)
A test that measures the number of blood cells in a blood sample. It includes the number of white blood cells, red blood cells, and platelets.

computed tomography (CT) scan
A test that uses x-rays from many angles to make a picture of the inside of the body.

Words to know

corticosteroids
A class of drug used to reduce redness, swelling, and pain, but also to kill cancer cells.

diagnosis
An identification of an illness based on tests.

flow cytometry
A test that measures myeloma cells in the bone marrow.

fluorescence in situ hybridization (FISH)
A lab test that uses special dyes to look for abnormal changes in a cell's genes and chromosomes.

fracture
A crack or break in a bone.

free light chain
The unattached, shorter fragments of M-proteins that are made by myeloma cells.

gene mutation
An abnormal change in the coded instructions within cells.

heavy chain
The longer protein chain that is part of an antibody.

high-dose chemotherapy
An intensive drug treatment to kill cancer and disease-fighting cells so transplanted blood stem cells aren't rejected by the body.

hyperviscosity
A condition in which the blood becomes very thick because of too many proteins in the blood.

immunoglobulin
A protein that is made by plasma cells to help fight off infection. Also called an antibody.

light chain
The shorter protein chain that is part of an antibody.

light chain myeloma
A condition in which myeloma cells make only free light chains and no complete M-proteins.

local therapy
Treatment that affects only one specific area of the body.

lymphocyte
A type of white blood cell that helps to protect the body from infection.

magnetic resonance imaging (MRI)
A test that uses radio waves and powerful magnets to view parts of the inside of the body and how they're working.

maintenance treatment
Medicine that's given in a lower dose or less often to keep (maintain) good results of prior treatments.

M-protein
An abnormal antibody made by myeloma cells that doesn't fight germs. Also called monoclonal protein.

mutation
An abnormal change in the genetic code (DNA) of a gene within cells.

observation
A period of testing for changes in cancer status while not receiving treatment.

pathologist
A doctor who's an expert in testing cells and tissue to find disease.

plasma cell
A type of white blood cell that makes germ-fighting proteins.

plasmacytoma
A mass formed by abnormal plasma cells (myeloma cells).

Words to know

positron emission tomography (PET)
A test that uses radioactive material to see the shape and function of organs and tissues inside the body.

primary treatment
The main treatment used to rid the body of cancer.

prognosis
The likely or expected course and outcome of a disease.

progression
The growth or spread of cancer after being tested or treated.

radiation therapy
A treatment that uses high-energy rays (radiation) to destroy cancer cells.

relapse
The return of myeloma signs or symptoms after a period of improvement.

side effect
An unhealthy or unpleasant physical or emotional response to treatment.

smoldering myeloma
Myeloma that isn't causing symptoms or damaging organs.

solitary plasmacytoma
Cancer that is one mass of myeloma cells.

stem cell transplant
Treatment that uses chemotherapy to destroy cells in the bone marrow and then replaces them with healthy blood stem cells.

supportive care
Treatment for symptoms of cancer or for the side effects of cancer treatment.

systemic therapy
Drugs used to treat cancer cells throughout the body.

targeted therapy
A drug treatment that targets a specific or unique feature of cancer cells.

tumor burden
A measure of the extent or amount of cancer in the body.

white blood cell
A type of blood cell that fights infection.

NCCN Contributors

This patient guide is based on the NCCN Clinical Practice Guidelines in Oncology (NCCN Guidelines®) for Multiple Myeloma, Version 3.2022. It was adapted, reviewed, and published with help from the following people:

Dorothy A. Shead, MS
Senior Director
Patient Information Operations

Rachael Clarke
Senior Medical Copyeditor

Tanya Fischer, MEd, MSLIS
Medical Writer

Laura J. Hanisch, PsyD
Program Manager
Patient Information Operations

Stephanie Helbling, MPH, MCHES®
Medical Writer

Susan Kidney
Senior Graphic Design Specialist

John Murphy
Medical Writer

Jeanette Shultz
Patient Guidelines Coordinator

Erin Vidic, MA
Medical Writer

Kim Williams
Creative Services Manager

NCCN Clinical Practice Guidelines in Oncology (NCCN Guidelines®) for Multiple Myeloma, Version 3.2022 were developed by the following NCCN Panel Members:

*Shaji K. Kumar, MD/Chair
Mayo Clinic Cancer Center

*Natalie S. Callander, MD/Vice Chair
University of Wisconsin Carbone Cancer Center

Kehinde Adekola, MD, MSCI
Robert H. Lurie Comprehensive Cancer Center of Northwestern University

Larry D. Anderson, Jr., MD, PhD
UT Southwestern Simmons Comprehensive Cancer Center

*Muhamed Baljevic, MD
Fred & Pamela Buffett Cancer Center

Erica Campagnaro, MD
University of Michigan Rogel Cancer Center

Jorge J. Castillo, MD
Dana-Farber/Brigham and Women's Cancer Center | Massachusetts General Hospital Cancer Center

Caitlin Costello, MD
UC San Diego Moores Cancer Center

Srinivas Devarakonda, MD
The Ohio State University Comprehensive Cancer Center - James Cancer Hospital and Solove Research Institute

Noura Elsedawy, MD
St. Jude Children's Research Hospital/ The University of Tennessee Health Science Center

Matthew Faiman, MD, MBA
Case Comprehensive Cancer Center/ University Hospitals Seidman Cancer Center and Cleveland Clinic Taussig Cancer Institute

Alfred Garfall, MD
Abramson Cancer Center at the University of Pennsylvania

Kelly Godby, MD
O'Neal Comprehensive Cancer Center at UAB

Jens Hillengass, MD, PhD
Roswell Park Comprehensive Cancer Center

Leona Holmberg, MD, PhD
Fred Hutchinson Cancer Research Center/ Seattle Cancer Care Alliance

Myo Htut, MD
City of Hope National Medical Center

Carol Ann Huff, MD
The Sidney Kimmel Comprehensive Cancer Center at Johns Hopkins

Malin Hultcrantz, MD, PhD
Memorial Sloan Kettering Cancer Center

Yubin Kang, MD
Duke Cancer Institute

Sarah Larson, MD
UCLA Jonsson Comprehensive Cancer Center

Michaela Liedtke, MD
Stanford Cancer Institute

Thomas Martin, MD
UCSF Helen Diller Family Comprehensive Cancer Center

*James Omel, MD
Patient Advocate

*Douglas Sborov, MD, MSc
Huntsman Cancer Institute at the University of Utah

Kenneth Shain, MD, PhD
Moffitt Cancer Center

Keith Stockerl-Goldstein, MD
Siteman Cancer Center at Barnes-Jewish Hospital and Washington University School of Medicine

Donna Weber, MD
The University of Texas MD Anderson Cancer Center

NCCN Staff

Rashmi Kumar, PhD

Ryan Berardi, MSc

* Reviewed this patient guide. For disclosures, visit NCCN.org/disclosures.

NCCN Cancer Centers

Abramson Cancer Center
at the University of Pennsylvania
Philadelphia, Pennsylvania
800.789.7366 • pennmedicine.org/cancer

Fred & Pamela Buffett Cancer Center
Omaha, Nebraska
402.559.5600 • unmc.edu/cancercenter

Case Comprehensive Cancer Center/
University Hospitals Seidman Cancer
Center and Cleveland Clinic Taussig
Cancer Institute
Cleveland, Ohio
800.641.2422 • UH Seidman Cancer Center
uhhospitals.org/services/cancer-services
866.223.8100 • CC Taussig Cancer Institute
my.clevelandclinic.org/departments/cancer
216.844.8797 • Case CCC
case.edu/cancer

City of Hope National Medical Center
Los Angeles, California
800.826.4673 • cityofhope.org

Dana-Farber/Brigham and
Women's Cancer Center |
Massachusetts General Hospital
Cancer Center
Boston, Massachusetts
617.732.5500
youhaveus.org
617.726.5130
massgeneral.org/cancer-center

Duke Cancer Institute
Durham, North Carolina
888.275.3853 • dukecancerinstitute.org

Fox Chase Cancer Center
Philadelphia, Pennsylvania
888.369.2427 • foxchase.org

Huntsman Cancer Institute
at the University of Utah
Salt Lake City, Utah
800.824.2073
huntsmancancer.org

Fred Hutchinson Cancer
Research Center/Seattle
Cancer Care Alliance
Seattle, Washington
206.606.7222 • seattlecca.org
206.667.5000 • fredhutch.org

The Sidney Kimmel Comprehensive
Cancer Center at Johns Hopkins
Baltimore, Maryland
410.955.8964
www.hopkinskimmelcancercenter.org

Robert H. Lurie Comprehensive
Cancer Center of Northwestern
University
Chicago, Illinois
866.587.4322 • cancer.northwestern.edu

Mayo Clinic Cancer Center
Phoenix/Scottsdale, Arizona
Jacksonville, Florida
Rochester, Minnesota
480.301.8000 • Arizona
904.953.0853 • Florida
507.538.3270 • Minnesota
mayoclinic.org/cancercenter

Memorial Sloan Kettering
Cancer Center
New York, New York
800.525.2225 • mskcc.org

Moffitt Cancer Center
Tampa, Florida
888.663.3488 • moffitt.org

The Ohio State University
Comprehensive Cancer Center -
James Cancer Hospital and
Solove Research Institute
Columbus, Ohio
800.293.5066 • cancer.osu.edu

O'Neal Comprehensive
Cancer Center at UAB
Birmingham, Alabama
800.822.0933 • uab.edu/onealcancercenter

Roswell Park Comprehensive
Cancer Center
Buffalo, New York
877.275.7724 • roswellpark.org

Siteman Cancer Center at Barnes-
Jewish Hospital and Washington
University School of Medicine
St. Louis, Missouri
800.600.3606 • siteman.wustl.edu

St. Jude Children's Research Hospital/
The University of Tennessee
Health Science Center
Memphis, Tennessee
866.278.5833 • stjude.org
901.448.5500 • uthsc.edu

Stanford Cancer Institute
Stanford, California
877.668.7535 • cancer.stanford.edu

UC Davis
Comprehensive Cancer Center
Sacramento, California
916.734.5959 • 800.770.9261
health.ucdavis.edu/cancer

UC San Diego Moores Cancer Center
La Jolla, California
858.822.6100 • cancer.ucsd.edu

UCLA Jonsson
Comprehensive Cancer Center
Los Angeles, California
310.825.5268 • cancer.ucla.edu

UCSF Helen Diller Family
Comprehensive Cancer Center
San Francisco, California
800.689.8273 • cancer.ucsf.edu

University of Colorado Cancer Center
Aurora, Colorado
720.848.0300 • coloradocancercenter.org

University of Michigan
Rogel Cancer Center
Ann Arbor, Michigan
800.865.1125 • rogelcancercenter.org

The University of Texas
MD Anderson Cancer Center
Houston, Texas
844.269.5922 • mdanderson.org

University of Wisconsin
Carbone Cancer Center
Madison, Wisconsin
608.265.1700 • uwhealth.org/cancer

UT Southwestern Simmons
Comprehensive Cancer Center
Dallas, Texas
214.648.3111 • utsouthwestern.edu/simmons

Vanderbilt-Ingram Cancer Center
Nashville, Tennessee
877.936.8422 • vicc.org

Yale Cancer Center/
Smilow Cancer Hospital
New Haven, Connecticut
855.4.SMILOW • yalecancercenter.org

Index

active (symptomatic) myeloma 10, 14, 24, 36, 44–48, 50

adjunctive treatment 39, 44, 48–49

allogeneic stem cell transplant 26, 35, 52

aspiration 20–21, 50

autologous stem cell transplant 35–36, 47–48, 50–51

biopsy 20–21, 45, 50

bisphosphonate 39–40, 48–49

blood clots 11, 31, 41, 49

blood stem cell 35–36, 42, 50

blood tests **10,** 17–18, 26, 46, 50

chemotherapy 12, 17, 29–33, 35–36, 47–48, 50, 55

clinical trial 10, 12, 29, 35, 37–38, 44, 46, 52, 55

gene 8, 22–23, 34

kidney damage 7, 10–12, 19–20, 26, 39, 40, 45, 49,

magnetic resonance imaging (MRI) 25, 50

maintenance treatment 26

M-protein 10–13, 18, 33, 39, 41, 45–46, 48

myeloma cell 10–13, 15, 17–18, 20–22, 25, 28, 30, 32, 34, 37, 39–40, 46, 48

PET/CT scan 24–25, 50

plasma cell 8–9, 13, 21, 26, 45–46, 50, 52

plasmacytoma 7, 34, 44–46

primary treatment 35, 39, 44, 46–51

progressive disease 44, 46, 50–52

radiation therapy 12, 32, 34, 40, 46, 49

relapse 30, 36, 47, 50–52

side effect 17, 29–32, 34, 36–37, 39, 41, 48–49, 51–52, 55

smoldering myeloma 10, 25, 44–45

stem cell transplant 12, 26, 29, 35–36, 47–48, 50–52

supportive care 35, 39, 41, 44, 47–49, 56

surgery 32, 34, 39–40, 46, 49, 55

targeted therapy 12, 17, 30–31, 48

treatment response 50–51

urine tests 18, 23, 45

Made in the USA
Middletown, DE
23 December 2021